Phonological disability in children

INGRAM

PHONOLOGICAL DISABILITY IN CHILDREN

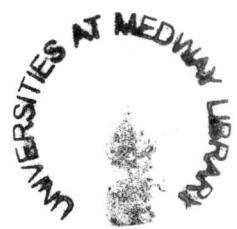

STUDIES IN DISORDERS OF COMMUNICATION

SECOND EDITION

W

WHURR PUBLISHERS
LONDON   JERSEY CITY

© Whurr Publishers Limited 1989

First published 1976 by
Edward Arnold (Publishers) Ltd
Reprinted 1990, 1992 and 1995 by Whurr Publishers Limited
19b Compton Terrace, London N1 2UN

British Library Cataloguing in Publication Data
Ingram, David, *1944–*
　Phonological disability in children.—
　2nd ed.
　1. Children. Language disorders
　I. Title　　II. Series
　618.92′855

ISBN 1–871381–05–3

Printed and bound by Antony Rowe Ltd, Eastbourne

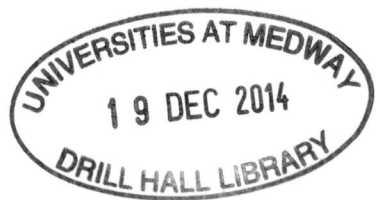

Contents

To Charles A. Ferguson

General preface

This series is the first to approach the problem of language disability as a single field. It attempts to bring together areas of study which have traditionally been treated under separate headings, and to focus on the common problems of analysis, assessment and treatment which characterize them. Its scope therefore includes the specifically linguistic aspects of the work of such areas as speech therapy, remedial teaching, teaching of the deaf and educational psychology, as well as those aspects of mother-tongue and foreign-language teaching which pose similar problems. The research findings and practical techniques from each of these fields can inform the others, and we hope one of the main functions of this series will be to put people from one profession into contact with the analogous situations found in others.

It is therefore not a series about specific syndromes or educationally narrow problems. While the orientation of a volume is naturally towards a single main area, and reflects an author's background, it is editorial policy to ask authors to consider the implications of what they say for the fields with which they have not been primarily concerned. Nor is this a series about disability in general. The medical, social, educational and other factors which enter into a comprehensive evaluation of any problems will not be studied as ends in themselves, but only in so far as they bear directly on the understanding of the nature of the language behaviour involved. The aim is to provide a much needed emphasis on the description and analysis of language as such, and on the provision of specific techniques of therapy or remediation. In this way, we hope to bridge the gap between the theoretical discussion of 'causes' and the practical tasks of treatment—two sides of language disability which it is uncommon to see systematically related.

Despite restricting the area of disability to specifically linguistic matters—and in particular emphasizing problems of the production and comprehension of spoken language—it should be clear that the series' scope goes considerably beyond this. For the first books, we have selected topics which have been particularly neglected in recent years, and which seem most able to benefit from contemporary research in linguistics and its related disciplines, English studies, psychology, sociology and education. Each volume will put its subject-matter in perspective, and will provide an introductory slant to its presentation. In this way, we hope to provide specialized studies which can be used as texts for components of teaching courses, as well as material that is directly applicable to the needs of professional workers. It is also hoped that this orientation will place the series within the reach of the interested layman—in particular, the parents or family of the linguistically disabled.

David Crystal
Jean Cooper

Preface

There is a delicate balance between personal interest and social need that has to be maintained each time an author takes on the important responsibility of writing a book. This is often forgotten in the commonplace statement that a book was written because there was a need for it. If one uses need in the sense of a lack of other works of exactly the same treatment, then indeed most books do satisfy a need. The need in these cases, however, is homogeneous with the research interests of the author. This may lead (although not inevitably so) to books on such specialized topics that they are only of interest to a handful of experts in the area.

This point was an important part of my decision to write a book on phonological disability in children instead of several other possible topics. This area is one of several that I find of great personal interest, yet I would be hard put to select one over another on that basis alone. Other social factors, however, enter into the decision. The first is the concern for practical application. In recent years, the progress made in the study of normal language acquisition has provided some exciting prospects in applying these findings to children with language disorders. As the quotation from Piaget at the beginning of this book so beautifully puts it, 'the mark of theoretical fertility in a science is its capacity for practical application.' While the theoretical work needs to continue, we have accumulated enough knowledge to allow application to be developed.

Even once this decision is made, there is still the problem of selecting the area to focus upon. Phonology was chosen for several reasons. For one thing, practical work in deviant phonology is currently behind that in the area of syntax in terms of availability to the public. At least two excellent books have already appeared on syntax, those of Tyack and Gottsleben (1974) and Crystal, Fletcher and Garman (1976). In addition, the articles available on phonology are often diverse and theoretical, making it difficult for clinicians to see their practical application. There is currently a gap between the rich and growing corpus of knowledge about both deviant and normal phonological development and the daily needs of language clinicians working with children who have phonological disorders.

The present book is an attempt to bridge this gap. As such, it is written specifically for language clinicians instead of linguists and psychologists, although I hope it will also be of interest to the latter. I have used a minimum of technical linguistic terminology and have tried whenever possible to define basic terms. Each chapter is designed to focus on an issue of specific interest to clinicians. The first chapter provides background information on the history of the study of child phonology, and addresses the all-important question of the potential contribution and limitation of linguistics. Next, there is an important chapter that outlines the development of phonology in normal children. This is needed in order to understand the process and compare it with aspects of development in deviant children. It is a long chapter because there is currently no book on normal child phonology. Since the key to clinical work is to be able to analyse the speech of children, chapter 3 provides a phonological analysis of a deviant child's speech. This is done to provide a model against which the clinician can compare his or her own analysis. The next chapter deals with the methodological issues of sampling, phonetic transcription, and testing. The last two chapters turn specifically to theoretical and practical questions. Chapter 5 provides a detailed comparison of the phonological characteristics of deviant speech with those of normal children, based on data available in the literature. It approaches the question of what constitutes deviant phonology. The last chapter directly discusses therapy and the application of the findings set out in earlier chapters. It also evaluates some hypotheses that have been proposed in the literature. As Piaget advises, throughout the book 'facts take precedence over theory.'

It would of course be impossible to acknowledge everyone who has contributed either directly or indirectly to the writing of this book. By far the most influential person has been Charles Ferguson, to whom it is dedicated. His contribution has been multidimensional. As my professor at Stanford University, he introduced me to child language in general and child phonology in particular—he has an international reputation in both. Since the completion of my PhD he has continued to stimulate my ideas through discussions and his papers on child phonology. From the beginning, he has taught me the importance of the need for practical application in linguistics, and the necessity to acquire facts before constructing theory. In the summer of 1974 he organized a seminar on deviant child phonology at Stanford University at which I taught, and which I used as the preparation for this book. It was one of the few applied courses of its kind ever offered in a linguistics programme. I would like to thank the many people I have met through the Institute for Childhood Aphasia who have helped me to understand better the various aspects of language disorders in children, especially Don Morehead, Jon Eisenson, Judith Johnston, Dee Tyack, Bill Rosenthal and Bob Gottsleben. I have benefited from conversations on deviant phonology from Mary Edwards, Kim Oller, and Arthur Compton. I owe a special appreciation to the members of the seminar I taught at Stanford, who helped me in many ways—Debbie Bresler, Tony Gillespie, Marcy Macken, Jan Moyers, Susan Payne, Irene Vogel and Brendan Webster. Lastly, two others have had a direct and immediate role in the writing—Judith Ingram, who read the book and straightened out many convoluted sentences (the responsibility for all that remain is my own), and David Crystal, joint editor of the series in which it appears, who arranged for its publication, provided editorial revision, and has in general continued to demonstrate a serious commitment to making linguistics socially responsible.

Preface to the Second Edition

In the Preface to the original edition to this book, I stated that a primary reason behind my undertaking such a task was to bring together in one place a range of ideas on both the theoretical and applied aspects of phonological disability. It has been my pleasant experience over the years since the book appeared to see the stimulus that it has been to research in this area. In the years shortly after, there were several works devoted to the assessment of phonological disorders in children. It is now commonplace for language clinicians to discuss in a sophisticated manner the phonological systems of the children which they treat. In fact, it may even be true that the assessment and remediation of children with phonological disability has surpassed that for syntax in terms of its accuracy and effectiveness.

In this second edition of the work, I have added an additional chapter which expresses some of the developments in my own thinking that have taken place since the original work. These developments are both in the area of explanation and that of methodology. Regarding theory, I outline some general ideas on the nature of normal phonological acquisition, and then make a simple hypothesis about the nature of phonological disability. The discussion of methodology deals with some advances since the discussion of this topic in Chapter 4. In large part, these ideas build upon, rather than replace, those in the original text. In addition, I have added a brief introduction to phonology in general at the onset of the new chapter. Those readers who lack a background in phonology may wish to begin with that section.

In addition to the acknowledgements to the original, I would like to mention some additional people who have influenced me greatly in more recent years. In the area of phonological disorders, I hold a special debt to discussions with and readings of research by Pamela Grunwell, Larry Leonard, John Locke, Richard Schwartz, and Carol Stoel-Gammon. The development of my theoretical views on normal acquisition has been aided greatly by discussions with Jane Fee, Heather Goad, and Cliff Pye. I would like to acknowledge a special debt to David Crystal, a remarkable linguist who has led the way for all of us who have attempted to bridge the gap between linguistics and language disorders in children. Lastly, I would like to mention the special importance of my friendship with Truman Coggins. I think that he, as much as anyone, has shown me how much research in the field of language disorders is driven by a deep caring for the children it helps.

Notation

The symbols presented below attempt to explain the wide range of notation used throughout the text. Since data have been cited from a variety of sources, there are occasional cases of different symbols for the same phonetic event. To capture this, I have placed alternant symbols in parentheses next to the more commonly used ones. Also, the use of various diacritics differs from one investigator to another. Thus the diacritics constitute a composite list rather than a set of consistent symbols used throughout.

Vowel symbols

	Front		Central	Back	
	unround	round		unround	round
high	i (iy)	ü		ɨ	u (uw)
	ɪ				ʊ
mid	e (ey)	ö (ø)			o (ow)
	ɛ		ə		ɔ
			ʌ		
low	æ			a	

Examples of English vowels

i	feet, meat, bee
ɪ	pit, fiddle, kid
e	may, plate, gate
ɛ	bet, pet, better
æ	cat, latin, fat
ə	sofa, about, telephone
ʌ	but, fun, butter
u	food, two, coo
ʊ	foot, would, put
o	goat, low, throw
ɔ	ball, saw, fought
ɑ	hot, bomb

Diphthongs

ay (ai) (aj)	bite, fight, light
æw	cow, how, house
ɔy	boy

Consonant Symbols

		Positions (*see below*)							
		1	2	3	4	5	6	7	8
Stops	vl	p			t			k	ʔ
	vd	b			d			g	
Affricates	vl				ts	č			
	vd				dz	ǰ			
Fricatives	vl	ø	f	θ	s	š(ʃ)		x	h
	vd	β	v	ð	z	ž		ɣ	ɦ
lateral					ɬ				
Nasals		m			n		ɲ	ŋ	
Liquids					l, r				
Glides		w					y		

vl = voiceless
vd = voiced

Positions

1 = labial	4 = alveolar	7 = velar
2 = labiodental	5 = alveopalatal	8 = glottal
3 = dental	6 = palatal	

Examples of English consonants

p	pit, paper, cap
b	bad, baby, cab
t	top, teeth, cot
d	do, bending, candied
k	cot, cap, kick
g	go, finger, fog
č	church, chip, catch
ǰ	jump, legion, fudge
f	foot, phone, cough
v	veal, fever, leave
θ	thick, ether, teeth

ð   the, father, bathe

s   soap, recent, face

z   zoo, razor, goes

š   shoe, wish, ration

ž   rouge, measure

m   money, mink, mop

n   no, many, man

ŋ   ring, think, singer

l   leave, lily, call

r   rope, mary, car

w   win, rowing

y   yes, yellow

Syllabic consonants

l̩   bottle, fiddle

r̩   bird, paper

m̩   bottom

n̩   button

Diacritic symbols

v́ or 'cv	before syllable indicates stress, e.g. bútter (or) 'butter
ṽ	nasal vowel
v: or v·	long vowel
v̆	short vowel
ç	voiceless consonant (used in some cases where a voiced consonant is only partially voiced)
cʰ or cʻ	aspirated consonant
ç	retroflexed consonant
c=	unaspirated consonant

Phonological symbols

C	consonant
V	vowel
[ ]	phonetic transcription
/ /	phonemic transcription, i.e. a sound unit that enters into contrast with others within the linguistic system

'Moreover, for teachers and all those whose work calls for an exact knowledge of the child's mind, facts take precedence over theory. I am convinced that the mark of theoretical fertility in a science is its capacity for practical application.'

Jean Piaget, *The language and thought of the child*

1

A linguistic approach

1.1 A growing interest in linguistics

In recent years there has been a growing emphasis on the role of linguistics in the field of language disorders in children. This phenomenon can partially be related to two recent developments in linguistics. The first of these is the appearance of transformational grammar with the publication of Noam Chomsky's *Syntactic structures* in 1957. This theory has provided an elegant and perceptive approach to language as well as powerful descriptive devices (e.g. transformations in the domain of syntax and distinctive features in phonology). Further, transformational grammar's emphasis on the need for linguistic theory to explain how children acquire linguistic structures has led to a renewed interest in language acquisition in children.

Both of these trends provide important new information in the area of language pathology. When confronted with children with language disorders, there is a need for a method of describing the child's linguistic system. This descriptive method must be effective in demonstrating the child's system of rules, and the complexity of the structures that are acquired. Some linguists feel that transformational grammar is a major step in this direction. When training children with language problems, it is also necessary to understand the general characteristics of the acquisition process. That is, one needs to know the various stages of language acquisition, on both general and specific topics, in order to determine any child's particular stage of arrest. Once determined, it is possible to see how far the child still needs to advance. Although these are worthy goals, it is not always clear to what extent each of these possible contributions has been incorporated directly into clinical application. To the working clinician, modern linguistics, especially transformational grammar, often appears to be a very theoretical and controversial approach to language. Since most linguists have not been concerned with matters of application they consequently have not made the appropriate adjustments to the theory. Also, those people who have attempted to make such modifications have often neglected the fact that others do not have the same experience in using linguistic methods of analysis. Their treatments are often advanced and outside the training of many clinicians. Lastly, it is not clear that many of the aspects of modern theory have direct clinical relevance, so that a realistic set of goals still needs to be established.

In terms of language acquisition in normal children, the same situation has developed to some extent. The claim is made that data on normal children can be invaluable to clinical work, yet a number of important questions remain to be answered. For example, although information is available on several aspects of normal language acquisition, it is generally not in a form that is readily adaptable for clinical evaluation and programming. Here, additional factors need to be considered, such as what to teach, how much, when, and how. The data on normal children are just a first step in such cases. Also, there is the ever-present question of the extent to which children with language disabilities follow the normal pattern. It may be that there are certain specific differences within individual disorders that will determine greatly how training should proceed.

These problems are particularly evident in the area of phonological disabilities in children. In the last few years there have been several articles discussing the value of generative (or transformational) approaches to phonological disability. The authors usually claim that they are providing an effective means to describe the phonological patterns of deviant children. Also, they claim that these descriptive devices, e.g. recent suggestions for the use of distinctive features, have therapeutic value. However, because of the assumptions made about the reader's linguistic background, these articles are often not understood by those concerned primarily with a clinical application. So, too, the conclusions drawn by the authors are often more theoretical than practical in scope. The result has been a rather negligible influence on most clinical practices.

To some extent, the same thing can be said about the use of data from normal children's phonological development. Apart from data on age norms for the appearance of particular sounds (e.g. Templin 1957), most normal data have not been adapted to clinical use. Often the information in diary studies is too sketchy or too detailed to provide a reasonable survey of the acquisition process. Other works often remain too theoretical or restricted in scope to provide information for application.

There is a tremendous need for a work which attempts to solve some of these problems. This is the general goal of this book. It approaches the topic of phonological disability from both the perspectives mentioned. In terms of phonological theory, it outlines those aspects of generative transformational theory that have direct clinical relevance. In doing so, a minimum of assumptions are made about the linguistic training of the reader. It is written for the language clinician who wishes to know how to better record, analyse, and programme the language of his or her children. In the process, data from normal as well as disabled children is presented and discussed to show how normal data may be used to improve clinical work with children.

1.2 The historical perspective

It is useful at the onset to take a brief look at the historical developments that have led to the existence of these two areas of information, i.e. phonological theory and data on normal children's phonological development.

1.21 Phonological theory

In terms of phonological theory, there are many alternative ways to look at the sound patterns of languages, and these alternatives vary considerably in the degree of support they receive from linguists throughout the world. For our purposes, two approaches are worth mentioning. The first approach is often called *taxonomic phonemics*, a term used to refer to a variety of approaches used extensively throughout the 1940s and 1950s. This approach is concerned with specifying the way languages use contrast to distinguish meanings in language. For example, English has /p/ and /b/ as contrasting sound units or *phonemes*, because the use of one or the other will cause a difference in meaning, e.g. *pit* versus *bit*. Relying on this principle, the area of taxonomic phonemics developed a number of assumptions about language and its analysis. The term 'taxonomic' is used because of the emphasis on classification.

With the advent of transformational grammar in the 1950s (also referred to as 'generative grammar'), a new approach to phonology was developed. This has come to be known as *generative phonology*, which differs from taxonomic phonemics in many ways. It was developed most extensively by the American linguists Noam Chomsky and Morris Halle, who in 1968 published the most extensive explanation yet of this theory in *The sound pattern of English*. Although this book was produced as a progress report on the state of the theory at that time, it still remains the primary source of information on it. Unfortunately, because it is a very difficult book to read, containing some unusual ideas about the nature of English phonology, some misunderstandings have arisen concerning the claims and value of generative phonology. A simpler and clearer treatment of the theory has been written by Schane (1973). This is a relatively useful introduction to the area of generative phonology, and should produce a wider understanding of its nature.

Although the details of the nature of generative phonology are outside the purpose of this book, at least two aspects deserve mention here. One of these concerns the use of *features* in describing language, i.e. the practice of breaking sounds down into their various parts. For example, the generative phonologist does not refer to a sound such as [b] as simply one unit, but rather one that can be further divided into features such as [+ stop], [+ labial], [+ voiced] etc. This practice has been carried over into a variety of studies with both deviant and normal children. A second point concerns the various *formal devices* this theory uses to describe the sound patterns of language. These include restrictions on how rules are written and the ways that rules may follow one another. These formal devices are commonly encountered in recent articles in speech journals on the application of generative phonology.

These two developments in phonological theory, taxonomic phonemics and generative phonology, have each had an influence on theories of child phonology. A theory of child phonology that in some ways grew out of taxonomic phonemics is that of Jakobson (1968), entitled *Child language, aphasia, and phonological universals*. This short book, which is actually a translation of a much earlier original in German, presents one of the most powerful theories of child phonology to date. In it, Jakobson emphasizes the claim that children learn contrasts, not just individual sounds. Also, he tries to predict the order in which sounds are acquired by saying that the first sounds to appear are those of maximal contrast. For example, the first contrast is that of the maximally closed consonant [m] or [p], versus the maximally open vowel [a].

A recent theory which has developed out of generative phonology is that proposed by Stampe (1969). Calling his approach 'Natural Phonology', Stampe has stressed the rule behaviour of young children. Whereas Jakobson talks about the child's behaviour as almost independent of the adult language, Stampe emphasizes that the child is constantly attempting an adult word. The child is said to have a set of innate processes that simplify the adult target word. The child does not say [ma] for any adult word, but only one such as *mother*, where the simplifying processes would delete the unstressed syllable and reduce the vowel to [a]. Those interested in the details of these and other theories are referred to Ferguson and Garnica 1975. The approach to child phonology that will follow in chapter 2 combines the insights of both Jakobson and Stampe by emphasizing both processes and contrasts.

1.22   Data on phonological development

The study of language acquisition in children can be divided into three main historical periods, based on the dominant methodological approach of the time. These are the period of diary studies (1877–1929); the period of large sample studies (1930–57); and the period of linguistic studies (1958–present). Each period contains major sources of data on phonological development in children. The nature of the data, however, varies greatly from one to the other.

During the early years of language acquisition studies, the primary method of study was that of the *diary*. The observer, typically a parent or relation of the child, recorded on a day-by-day basis the speech of the child. This approach has continued to be used, improved in recent years by the availability of electronic recording equipment. Although there were several excellent phonological diaries during this period in other languages, this was not so for English. Instead, there were only a few sporadic studies that often did not report all the data collected. Some of the better ones include Hills 1914 and Humphreys 1880. Since this period other diaries have appeared, yet only two works, by Leopold (1947) and Smith (1973), qualify as major studies. Leopold observed his daughter Hildegard during the earliest period, following her development from the first words until the age of two. Smith observed the phonology of his son longitudinally between the ages of two and four. Each provides data on different periods of development. The advantage of studies such as these lies especially in the raw data they provide, allowing others to pursue analyses of their own.

In the area of phonological disability in children, diary accounts are virtually nonexistent. During the entire diary period the only study providing extensive data on a delayed child is that of Hinckley (1915). The transcription, however, was less than satisfactory. Recent studies on the phonology of various children with disorders do not qualify as diary studies. They rarely present the data collected or provide longitudinal observations, an unfortunate state of affairs. This gap of information is one of the major reasons for much of our ignorance in this area of study. It is to be hoped that this will be corrected by future work.

The second period of studies can be dated from 1930 with the publication of Dorothea McCarthy's book *Language development of the preschool child*, which initiated a number of studies designed to gather information on large numbers of children. In many ways, this was the exact opposite of the diary study. Instead of extensive data from a single child, short samples of speech from large numbers of children across different ages were collected. During the diary study period, there was some interest in making claims about acquisition across children (e.g. the studies by Tracy 1893 and Lukens 1894), but these were rather unsystematic, based on collected diary accounts. The large sample studies elicited specific, target sounds.

In the domain of normal children's phonology, there are three major studies of this sort. The first was by Wellman *et al.* (1931), entitled 'Speech sounds of young children'. They elicited English speech sounds from 215 children between 1;6 (one year, six months) and 6;6. These results, like all of this sort, were quantitatively presented in terms of percentages of correct use per age group, providing the first guidelines as to when specific speech sounds are acquired. This study was followed by one by Poole (1934), a dissertation which unfortunately has only been published in abstract form. She studied 140 children from 2;6 to 8;6. The best study of this kind was by Templin, who in 1957 published *Certain language skills in children*. Part of this monograph is an articulation study of 480 children between 3 and 8 years of age in which Templin elicited 176 sounds and sound combinations from each child. Her results still represent the norm against which most children are compared. Winitz 1969 provides a survey and comparison of these three studies. Recently, a large sample study by Olmsted (1971) has appeared. Olmsted collected spontaneous speech from 100 children between 1;3 and 4;6. Like those before him, his study is by and large quantitative, although he has developed different measures of acquisition from the simple percentages of correct use found in the others.

A few large sample studies have been attempted on the phonology of deviant children. Bangs (1942) studied the articulatory defects of 53 mentally retarded subjects. He provides a quantitative analysis of the main substitutions, omissions and additions in their speech elicited through picture cards. Hudgins and Numbers (1942) did the most extensive study of this kind, reporting on the phonological patterns of 192 deaf pupils between 8 and 20 years old. A third and more recent study is that of Morley (1957), who gives the major substitution patterns used by children with language disorders.

Since 1957 there has been a marked change in the approach to the study of children's language. This change has been towards more linguistic analyses of the language of children. That is, instead of only looking at the output of the child, there is an insistence on determining the rule behaviour behind that output as well. Studies of this kind are constantly referring to the *rules* that children use to produce language, and how these rules change in time. In the area of child phonology, this has led to studies which go beyond the general notion of substitution used before. Previously, much was made of listing the sounds the child had and noting substitutions that occurred for adult ones. Now, the emphasis has shifted to noting the rules behind these substitutions. For example, instead of saying that the child uses the substitutions [b] for [v], [d] for [z], [d] for [ð], the three are said to be one rule or process which makes voiced fricatives into stops. Some recent studies of the speech of normal children that fall under this approach include those of Menn (1971), Moskowitz (1970), Kornfeld (1971), Waterson (1971), Smith (1973) and Ingram (1974a).

This approach has also dominated the most recent work in the area of phonological disability. Research has taken several directions, but each study has shown a commitment to the use of linguistic methodology, specifically looking for general rule-based behaviour. One type has been largely descriptive, concerned with presenting a *case study* or studies of children with disorders in articulation. These include studies by Haas (1963), Oller *et al.* (1972), West and Weber (1973), Edwards and Bernhardt (1973), Oller and Kelly (1974), Bodine (1974) and Lorentz (1974). Others have been concerned specifically with demonstrating the utility of linguistics in the analysis and remediation of phonological disorders. These include studies by Crocker (1969), Compton (1970, 1975), McReynolds and Huston (1971), McReynolds and Bennett (1972), Pollock and Rees (1972) and Oller (1973).

In several ways, this book comes under this last category. It is basically an attempt to demonstrate the utility of linguistics in analysing and remediating the speech of children with articulation disorders. It results from the need for a treatment of the various suggestions and findings to date.

1.3 The contribution of linguistics

Suggestions are often made concerning the contribution of linguistics to speech pathology without ever justifying its use. What contributions has linguistics to offer to speech remediation, and what are its limitations? There are obviously contributions to be made; it is because of this that so many recent studies have appeared. At the same time, it is important at the outset to specify both the kind and variety of contributions possible, as well as the feasibility of their fulfilment at the present time. This has not always been done, which has occasionally led to misunderstanding, particularly through unrealistic claims for success.

An excellent article on this topic has recently been written by Crystal (1972). He outlines the kinds of contributions from linguistics that would be of value to the language clinician, their current state of achievement and their limitations. The following discussion is greatly influenced by his treatment, although it has been modified to deal specifically with the question of phonology. A presentation of these contributions will also be used to introduce the subject-matter of the following chapters.

What, then, are the contributions that linguistics can make to the language clinician who must deal with children with phonological disabilities? Stated differently, what set of books or materials could the linguist provide to the clinician for reference when needed? There are at least five major areas in which linguistics can contribute.

(*a*) First, there is the need for *general treatments of the topic of phonology*, specifically designed for nonlinguists. There are two areas that need to be covered. One is a general discussion of the basic principles of phonological theory, which can be found in general introductions to linguistics. Several sound introductions exist, two especially excellent ones being Crystal 1971, and Fromkin and Rodman 1974. The latter has a particularly good treatment of phonology. Also, one can turn to specific books on phonology. The best introduction to generative phonology to date is that by Schane (1973). A recent introduction to phonetics is O'Connor 1972.

Second, there is a need for a good introduction to the phonology of English. Such a book should outline the basic sound patterns of English, highlighting the occurrence of the various English phonemes and their permissible combinations. This would be a valuable reference source for the clinician. Crystal, in his article, suggests that Gimson 1970 satisfies this need.

(*b*) Besides knowledge of English phonology, it would be useful for the clinician to have a comprehensive book on *how normal children acquire English phonology*. Although our knowledge in this area has increased greatly since the days of the first diaries, there is currently no book that comes close to summarizing all that is known. The only books available on the acquisition of phonology are primarily either theoretical treatments or diary accounts. Because of this lack, chapter 2 will provide a general survey of phonological development in normal children.

(*c*) While all the above information is of great use to the clinician, there is still the practical issue of determining the nature of each child's phonological system. There is a need for *a set of techniques for the collection and analysis of children's speech*. Suggestions in these areas is spread throughout the various articles that have appeared in recent years. In the area of syntax, there are now available two sources of information in this regard—Tyack and Gottsleben 1974 and Crystal *et al.* 1976. Chapters 3 and 4 of this book will provide some techniques for phonology, beginning with phonological analysis in chapter 3. Data is presented from one child and analysed in a step-by-step fashion to determine the main phonological patterns of the child's system.

Besides analysis, there is also need for the presentation of techniques for the collection, transcription and recording of data from children for analysis. Linguistics has developed a number of procedures in this area. Some of the issues involved here include ways to elicit speech samples, methods of taperecording, systems of phonetic transcription, the need for more than one transcriber, and the format for organizing data for record-keeping. A true picture of a child's progress can be obtained only after accurate samples of speech are gathered at predetermined intervals. Chapter 4 deals with the techniques needed to collect and record phonological samples.

(*d*) A fourth contribution of linguistics would be a book characterizing the *nature of phonological disability in children*. There are several questions that must be answered in this regard. Do children with articulation difficulties nonetheless show systematic substitutions and processes in their speech? If so, are the processes the same as those used by normal children, and if not, how do they differ? Do the processes differ according to the particular disorder? For example, do children who are retarded show different phonologies from those who are hard of hearing? At present we only have partial answers to these questions. Chapter 5 deals with each in turn, in the light of current knowledge.

(*e*) Even if all this information were available, there would still be the major problem that confronts each therapist, day after day: the remediation of the child. What does all this information mean when it comes down to assisting the child in overcoming his or her speech impediment? Here there is need for a *set of principles for the planning of therapy*. These principles, based on how children acquire phonology, must be able to predict what will be easiest for the child to learn, given the current status of his or her language. They also should outline how this may most effectively be taught. In this regard Crystal (1972) has said, 'The linguist cannot yet answer with any confidence the question "what structure should I teach next?", but he can offer good advice about the range of structures available, and this in itself is useful, for one can make a wise choice only when one knows the alternatives' (15).

Chapter 6 will discuss several of the approaches currently being proposed in the area of remediation. As Crystal advises, these are not presented as dogma to be followed to the letter, but as available alternatives to the more simplistic approach of teaching sound by sound, with the only goal being immediate correct production. Some of the issues that need to be addressed include: the elimination of general processes rather than individual substitution; the question of generalization, where one sound is taught with the expectation that other, similar sounds will change; the teaching of phonemic contrasts within the child's own system rather than just those of the adult language; and ways to determine which sounds to teach first. The data for and against each approach will be evaluated. In this area, linguistics can provide some interesting and provocative suggestions for remediation that can subsequently be subjected to empirical investigation. It is here that Crystal (1972) sees the prime contribution of linguistics, which is 'as an aid in the development of a *more explicitly principled therapy*' [italics mine] (3).

1.4 The limitations of linguistics

Just as there are areas where linguistics can assist the clinician in remediating the language of children, there are also several limitations to these contributions. That is, linguistics is by no means an answer to every problem faced by the clinician. Crystal points out several limitations in his excellent discussion.

The goals and interests of phonological theory differ in many ways from those of the clinician. The clinician who turns to it to acquire information for his or her practice will be confronted with numerous issues that are of no interest. For example, there are various phonological theories, and much of phonological study is devoted to theoretical arguments for or against each. Also, there is usually a strong concern for formalism. The emphasis on theory and formal issues are often obscure exercises to the clinician who has to deal daily with very practical matters. In addition, phonology concerns itself with all languages, not just English.

To overcome this, either programmes of instruction need to be developed which focus on those areas of phonology of immediate use to clinicians, or else general courses should be taught by linguists who are aware of the clinician's practical needs. This, however, leads to a second limitation of linguistics. Most linguists have been trained in programmes that emphasize theoretical issues over more practical ones. This has been effectively pointed out by Newmeyer and Emonds (1971). As a result, most linguists are essentially insensitive to the practical needs of the clinician. Fortunately, more linguists are becoming concerned about this dilemma. In the meantime, however, the clinician should be aware of this attitude in some linguists. This lack of experience has led to misunderstandings between the two disciplines. The linguist often has little understanding of the problems and interests of the clinician; the clinician often has difficulty understanding the theoretical concerns of the linguist. As long as these differences in interest exist, there will be a limitation on the contribution of linguistics.

Another limitation of linguistics is the fact that many of the problems confronted by the clinician are nonlinguistic problems, such as the emotional state of the child, his behaviour and his relationship in the family. Language remediation is just one of several aspects which concern the clinician.

This book attempts to overcome the first two of these limitations. Regarding the first, the discussion on phonological theory is limited to that part which touches directly upon the question of acquisition by young children. It presupposes a minimum of background and avoids metatheoretical issues. Also, the emphasis on formalism is minimal, since much of the formal apparatus developed by linguists is not needed to analyse and characterize the child's speech effectively. In this way the book departs from some recent articles on the application of generative phonology to speech therapy which have emphasized formal devices.

To remedy the second point, this book deals primarily with practical issues. After presenting a survey of normal phonological acquisition, the book concentrates on matters specifically related to the nature of phonological disability in children. The focus turns to the collection and analysis of speech samples, the nature of deviant phonology, and issues in remediation. These are all issues that confront the clinician every day in his or her practice.

2

Aspects of phonological acquisition

2.1 The study of the normal child

It is certainly justifiable to ask at the onset whether or not the study of the normal child will benefit work with children with language disorders. One could even set up two extreme camps, one arguing that it is only necessary to look at normal children, the other saying that this never needs to be done. The arguments for each might run as follows: for the normal-centred group, the deviant child is simply a slowed-down version of the normal process of acquisition. Consequently, the study of the normal process provides all the information one needs. For the deviant-centred position, the abnormal process of acquisition is unique and merits independent study of its own. For this group, information on normal children would be of no interest.

It is easy to see that both these extremes are wrong, and that the study of both kinds of acquisition is in order. Data from normal children provide our basic knowledge about the process of acquisition and the norms against which others are compared. The comparison of the speech of language-disturbed children with that of normal children helps us to define what developmental processes are normal and which are not. Study to date suggests that in both syntax (Morehead and Ingram 1973) and phonology (Oller 1973), the deviant child shows many patterns similar to those of normal children. Knowledge of normal acquisition, then, provides the starting-point for the study of deviance.

Once this is done, it is necessary to study the speech of children with disorders. Despite the many similarities between the two groups, there are also individual and group differences. These will need to be uncovered and examined in detail. This can only be done through the collection of data from deviant children and comparison with normal processes. This chapter will focus on the acquisition of phonology in normal children. The question of what constitutes deviance will be treated in chapter 5.

2.2 Stages of phonological development

In studying acquisition, it is useful to have a general framework to work from. The best way to do this is to provide general stages of acquisition, and then look at each stage in detail. Thus, it is possible to place in a continuum any child in any stage of the acquisition process.

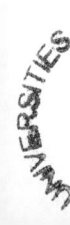

In terms of phonology, there has been virtually no research into the constructing of general stages of acquisition. In fact, this is more or less true also of grammatical development, where most proposals concerning stages deal with specific grammatical constructions rather than wider behaviour. Consequently, most statements about general stages are tentative and subject to further elaboration.

In examining stages of phonological development, it is possible to attempt a comparison with general stages of language. Indeed, as will be shown, it is even possible, and perhaps necessary, to make the comparison with cognitive stages of development. In this way, a greater picture of the child's progress is available.

The first issue in determining stages is to decide the beginning and the end of the process. In phonology it is often suggested that it starts with the first words at 1;6, and ends around age 6 or so, with the acquisition of the last, few troublesome speech sounds. In the meantime, the main advances take place from 2 to 4. Here, however, it is suggested that this development needs to be considered over a broader age range, specifically from birth to the sixteenth year at least. A framework that takes such a broad view of the child's development is available in the theory of Jean Piaget. Within Piaget's general stages of cognitive ability, one can see corresponding grammatical and phonological behaviours. These are displayed in table 1.

Table 1   Piaget's cognitive stages of development with approximate ages, and the grammatical and phonological stages that correspond to each

Piaget's stages	Linguistic stages	Phonological stages
Sensori-motor period (0;0–1;6) Development of systems of movements and perception. Child achieves notion of object permanence.	1 Prelinguistic communication through gestures and crying. 2 Holophrastic stage. Use of one-word utterances.	1 Prelinguistic vocalization and perception (birth to 1;0). 2 Phonology of the first 50 words (1;0–1;6).
Period of concrete operations (1;6–12;0) Preconcept subperiod (1;6–4;0) The onset of symbolic representation. Child can now refer to past and future, although most activity is in the here and now. Predominance of symbolic play.	3 Telegraphic stage. Child begins to use words in combinations. These increase to point between 3 and 4 when most sentences become close to well-formed, simple sentences.	3 Phonology of single morphemes. Child begins to expand inventory of speech sounds. Phonological processes that result in incorrect productions predominate until around age 4 when most words of simple morphological structure are correctly spoken.
Intuitional subperiod (4;0–7;0). Child relies on immediate perception to solve various tasks. Begins to develop the concept of reversibility. Child begins to be involved in social games.	4 Early complex sentences. Child begins to use complements on verbs and some relative clauses. These early complex structures, however, appear to be the result of juxtaposition.	4 Completion of the phonetic inventory. The child acquires production of troublesome sounds by age 7. Good production of simple words. Beginning of use of longer words.
Concrete operations subperiod (7;0–12;0). Child learns the notion of reversibility. Can solve tasks dealing with conservation of mass, weight, and volume.	5 Complex sentences. Child acquires the transformational rules that embed one sentence into another. Coordination of sentences decreases, v. the increase in complex sentences.	5 Morphophonemic development. Child learns more elaborate derivational structure of the language; acquires morphophonemic rules of language.
Period of formal operations (12;0–16;0). Child learns the ability to use abstract thought. Can solve problems through reflection.	6 Linguistic intuitions. Child can now reflect upon grammaticality of his speech and arrive at linguistic intuitions.	6 Spelling. Child masters ability to spell.

For a brief but valuable description of the Piagetian stages, the reader is referred to Piaget (1962, 273–91). There are also several introductions available, including Piaget and Inhelder 1969. It is worth pointing out, however, that familiarity with Piaget's theory is not a prerequisite to the present book. Rather, it is presented simply to place phonological development in relation to other aspects of human development.

The first major period of cognitive development is the Sensori-Motor Period which runs from birth to 1;6 to 2 years of age. During this time the infant develops its senses and motor skills, as well as its ability to imitate. The period ends with the child's attainment of the notion of the permanent object. The child realizes that it is but one of many objects with various shapes, dimensions and other characteristics. For Piaget, this is the period which precedes language, i.e. the use of arbitrary signs to communicate meaning.

During this period there are two stages involving linguistic development in general and phonological development in particular. First, there is the period of time before the child's first words, which runs from birth to around 10 months to one year of age. During this time the child communicates (first unintentionally and later intentionally) through crying and crude gestures. Several important prerequisite developments take place in preparation for phonological development. The ability to discriminate perceptually develops very rapidly. Several recent investigations have shown this in infants as young as one month (cf. the review of this research in Eimas 1974 and Morse 1974). This will later prove to be an important skill in identifying adult words. Also, the child enters into sound play, or babbling, which at later months will constitute some of the child's first words (e.g. *mama, baba* etc.). Related to this, the child also increases its ability to imitate. This follows several stages (to which I will return later) until a point at which the child can imitate new sounds, and also retain these for later 'deferred imitations'. Piaget has emphasized the important role the latter plays in the development of symbolic behaviour.

Secondly, the child enters the period of one-word utterances, which lasts from about 1;0 to 1;6. During this time the child acquires a small vocabulary until it reaches approximately 50 words about 1;6. At that time the end of the stage is marked by two behavioural changes—a sudden increase in vocabulary and the onset of two-word utterances. During at least the early part of the one-word utterance (or holophrastic, meaning one word = one sentence) stage, the child as yet does not have linguistic signs as we know them. Rather, Piaget notes that these early symbols are far from being socially recognized signs of reference, but rather constitute unstable, fleeting symbols of the child's world. Thus, a sound such as *bow-wow* may refer to a dog one day, a horse another, or even a clock the next, if the sound constitutes the current symbol of the child. This qualitative difference between the words of the holophrastic period and those after 1;6 and the onset of real linguistic signs is important with regard to phonology. In several ways the phonological aspects of the words during this time, which we can call the Phonology of the First 50 Words, is different from the developments which follow. It therefore constitutes a separate stage of acquisition that merits separate investigation.

The second period of cognitive development, the Period of Concrete Operations, covers an enormous span of time (1;6 or 2 to 11 or 12), and can be divided into three main subperiods. This period marks the onset of the ability of representation (i.e. to re-present reality through the use of linguistic signs) and thus the onset of language. During the three subperiods there are also analogous grammatical and phonological developments.

The first subperiod is that of Preconceptual Thought, lasting from 1;6 or 2 to

4 or 4;6. This is the first time when the child can develop the use of symbolic behaviour. As a result, there is a predominance of symbolic play, e.g. the practice that a block of wood constitutes a car, a leaf is a blanket, etc. The child is very much in the here and now during this time, using language to comment on his own activities and interests. Linguistically, this is the stage during which the child progresses from putting two words together to the point around 3;6 to 4;0 when most simple sentences are well formed by adult standards. Before this point, however, most utterances are incomplete, leading to their description under the general term of Telegraphic Stage (cf. Brown 1973 for a more precise breakdown of the linguistic stages of this period).

Phonologically, this is also a very active period of development. With the increase of vocabulary that marks the onset of this stage, the child is confronted with the first real necessity to develop a phonological system. From 1;6 on, the child enters the period of phonological development that is most commonly described in the literature. During this time, the child continues to add new sounds to his or her language, while still making a number of changes to adult words. It is a period marked by what parents refer to as cute forms, such as *goggie* for *doggie*, *tat* for *cat*, *shish* for *fish* etc. Later we will return to the kinds of processes that result in forms such as these. Finally, around age 4, the child has reasonable control over most of the sounds of English. The unfamiliar adult can usually recognize without difficulty the child's speech at this time. What remains ahead consists of two further achievements. First, the child still needs to master the last, lingering sounds that pose unusual articulation difficulties. This will often take another two or three years of practice. Second, the child has yet to acquire very complex words of English. Most of its vocabulary consists of simple two- or three-syllable words of a single morpheme. It is only later that accurate pronunciation includes more elaborate, morphologically complex forms. It is because of this that the achievements during this stage are limited to the phonology of simple morphemes.

The next cognitive step is the intuitional subperiod from around 4;0 to 6 or 7. During this stage, the child comes closer to an understanding of reality and begins to abandon the dominant use of symbolic play. Rather than modify reality through play, the child begins to use play to express reality. The child begins to enter into social games with other children, although she or he still does not accept that there are arbitrary, socially-accepted rules to them. Instead, he prefers to change the rules at will to his own momentary interests. In coming closer to reality, the child uses 'intuitions' to solve problems, these intuitions being based on the child's immediate perception of reality. Piaget refers to this as 'centration'. For example, when asked which of two containers has more water, the child will 'centre' on the height of the water, and intuit that the higher one must have more.

Linguistically, the child begins to use much more frequently a number of complex sentence structures. A variety of verb complements (e.g. 'John thinks *that Joe's silly*') and relative clauses (e.g. 'I like the boy *who's there*') become more frequent parts of the child's speech. At the same time, however, the child also predominantly uses coordination between sentences, e.g. 'I went home *and* I wanted to have a sandwich *and* I wanted to play.' An examination of children's texts at this age shows that many of these coordinations could be eliminated by embedding one of the sentences into the other. The above utterance, for example, could have been 'I went home to have a sandwich and play.' Consequently, it is not clear that the child as yet has a productive system of rules for sentence embedding. Rather, juxtaposition appears to be the dominant structural characteristic. So, just as cognitively the child begins to anticipate the concrete operations of the next stage through intuition, the child uses structures that anticipate the rule-based generation of complex sentences of the next stage.

In phonology, similar developments occur. First, the developments of the previous stage are refined. In syntax, simple sentences are now more or less well formed. So too, the phonological inventory is completed during this period. By the age of 7 most speech sounds are accurately acquired. In this sense, this is the time of the Completion of the Phonetic Inventory. Secondly, the child begins to use words that anticipate rule-based developments of the next stage. Specifically, the child begins to use more complex words that will require knowledge of morphophonemic alternations (e.g. changes such as *electric* > *electricity*, where the [k] becomes an [s]). The child will experiment with new words during this time, using them in a variety of contexts to try them out. It is not clear, though, that the child is aware of the phonological alternations required in these more complex words. This awaits the rapid growth of vocabulary and understanding of the next period.

The next subperiod, from 7;0 to 12;0, that of Concrete Operations, is an important stage of development cognitively. The child develops the ability to perform reversible operations, i.e. to go back and retrace events to solve various kinds of problems. The child learns how to 'transform' reality. In syntax, this also appears to be the time when children acquire many of the more complex structures of language. Passives, relative clauses etc. become more dominant parts of the child's system. It appears that the onset of reading has much to do with this development (cf. O'Donnell *et al.* 1967). Likewise, in phonology the child acquires the derivational morphology of the language. Here too, it seems that reading has something to do with this (Moskowitz 1973). The child, then, develops over these years the more complex aspects of his language.

About age 12, the child reaches the last of Piaget's three major Periods. This is the Period of Formal Operations, when the child becomes capable of abstract, reflective thought. The child no longer is tied to what is real and ongoing, but can reflect on both the possible and impossible. At this time, the child linguistically becomes capable of making intuitional reflections on his language. That is, he can think of what can be said and what cannot. Decisions of grammaticality can be made. In phonology, the child can also begin to decide what is a possible sound change and what is not. This probably also has an effect on spelling, which develops markedly during this period.

These then are the general stages that phonological development seems to follow. No doubt improvement and elaboration is needed, but they provide a useful framework in which one can place the developing child. The next section looks more closely at the phonological characteristics of each of these stages, with the major emphasis on those of the first four years, which are the most relevant to the problem of children with phonological disorders.

2.3 Some general phonological characteristics

The preceding section provides a survey of phonological development and its relationship to other aspects of development. Here we shall look in more detail at the characteristics of each of the preceding phonological stages.

2.31 Preverbal vocalization and perception

A very recent finding is that children in the first months of life show an ability to discriminate perceptually between fine differences between sounds. These studies are reviewed by Morse (1974) and Eimas (1974). This has been shown through the use of a habituation-dishabituation paradigm, where the child is presented a series of exposures to the same syllable, e.g. [ba, ba, ba] etc., and then suddenly presented a new syllable, e.g. [pa, pa, pa]. After hearing the first syllable constantly repeated, the child loses interest in it, i.e. becomes habituated. Then, if he has the ability to notice the new syllable, a dishabituation or renewed interest will result. These shifts of interest have been measured primarily through two response modes, heart rate and non-nutritive sucking (with a pacifier specifically wired to record the rate). The most convincing data (according to Morse 1974) has been in older infants (5 to 6 months), where [ba] versus [ga] has been discriminated. Studies with younger infants have had more varied results, but nonetheless are promising. No doubt the development of more sophisticated procedures in this area will lead to very interesting findings. So far, this research has concentrated on normal infants.

One important point to keep in mind in regard to these studies is that they do not deal with linguistic perception. That is, the children do not have to discriminate meaningful utterances. This is important because studies with children learning languages have shown that perception is far from perfect in the early stages. These studies will be presented below in Section 2.331. Despite this, it seems likely that this early ability to discriminate nonmeaningful speech is an important precursor of later linguistic development.

Before the first words, the child engages in a variety of sound production that is often called cooing or babbling. The term cooing is often restricted to the sounds made in the first four months or so which are largely vocalic with an increasing number of velar or back consonantal sounds. During the middle months of the first year, a shift occurs to more labial consonants, which marks the stage referred to as babbling. A functional difference is also occasionally made between the two. Cooing is said to be more directly linked to the expression of pleasure, whereas babbling seems more like sound play for its own sake, apart from an expression of bodily comfort. Most data on segmental development are based on Irwin 1947.

The description of babbling and its role in phonological development has been controversial. Jakobson (1968), for example, has argued that it plays no role in phonological development. He has also said that the child is capable of babbling all possible sounds. Despite the fact that both of these claims can be shown to be wrong, they still appear at times in introductory books on the topic. Irwin's research, as well as more recent work (e.g. Blount 1970), has shown that babbling is not as random as Jakobson suggests, and that a progression occurs. Also, the usefulness of babbling is not simply one of practice, but is interlinked with the entire process of learning to represent adult words. This can be seen through an examination of the stages of imitative ability in the first year and a half.

Piaget (1962) has emphasized the importance of imitation in the development of language. The child becomes capable of internalized imitation of speech sounds, no longer needing an immediate model to produce them. The stages of imitative ability and the role of the child's own vocalization (or babbling) can be seen in table 2. At some time during the first four months, the child will vocalize when

Table 2 Imitative ability during Piaget's sensori-motor stages, based on Piaget 1962

Sensori-motor Stage	Imitative ability Nonverbal	Verbal
I (0;0–0;1)		Cries when hears others cry.
II (0;1–0;4)	Sporadic imitation of movements by visible body parts.	Vocal contagion—vocalizes at the sound of the human voice imitating the child.
III (0;4–0;8)	Systematic imitation of movements child has already made and seen.	Imitates sounds that he can spontaneously make.
IV (0;8–1;0)	Imitation of movements already made by child but which are not visible.	First attempts at new sounds not yet made by child.
V (1;0–1;4)	Systematic imitation of new models not made by child, including those that are not visible to child.	First attempts to reproduce adult words. This is done through trial and error.
VI (1;4–1;6)	Deferred imitation of models seen earlier.	Deferred imitation of words heard earlier, e.g. child said 'in step' without ever having said it before.

the adult does. This vocal contagion or mutual imitation does not entail specific segments of speech. The adult, however, needs to make sounds similar to the child's own sounds to ensure vocalization. In the next stage, 4 to 8 months of age, the child begins to imitate specific sounds of the adult, but only if the sounds are similar to those made spontaneously by the child. The first attempts at new sounds occur between 8 to 12 months, followed by attempts to reproduce adult words in the first months of the second year. Deferred imitation makes the last and very important step in this process, the ability to retain a model for imitation at a later time. All these stages show a progression toward the onset of the first words of language, a progression tied to the child's imitative ability which in turn is linked to his own spontaneous vocalization. This is a very important part of Piaget's theory, the point that all development is built upon previous developments. In this sense, then, babbling is an important precursor to phonological development. Oller *et al.* (1974) have even suggested from preliminary findings of their own that children in their later speech show patterns similar to those used in their earlier babbling. If this is substantiated by further research, it is more evidence for the relation of babbling to later speech.

2.32   Phonology of the first 50 words

As already noted, the holophrastic stage of language acquisition lasts about six months, from approximately the first year to 1;6. During this period, the child comes to acquire about 50 words before his vocabulary begins to grow very rapidly (cf. Nelson 1973). The nature of the child's phonology is very primitive during this time, and can be discussed as a separate period of acquisition. Many of the studies of phonological development have focused on this eary stage.

The most famous description of acquisition for this period is in Jakobson 1968 and Jakobson and Halle 1956. Here, I will restrict the discussion to the facts Jakobson noted on the period. First, he found through surveying various diary accounts that children frequently show the same first sounds during this time. This led him to suggest that there is a universal order of acquisition. Generally, he found:

(a)   The first syllables are CV or CVCV reduplicated.
(b)   The first consonants are labial, most commonly [p] (or perhaps [m]).
(c)   These are followed by [t], and later [k].
(d)   The first vowel is [a], followed later by [i] and/or [u].
(e)   A homorganic fricative is acquired only if the stop has been acquired.

Ferguson and Garnica (1975) have also pointed out that Jakobson missed the following fact:

(f)   [h] and [w] are often among the first sounds acquired.

Table 3   First 25 recorded forms of four normal children, based on published diary information in Velten 1943, Menn 1971, Leopold 1947 and Ingram 1974a

Joan Velten	Daniel Menn*	Hildegard Leopold	Jennika Ingram
0;10	1;4	0;10	1;3
up [ap]	*byebye* [bab]	*pretty* [prɔti]	*blanket* [ba]
bottle [ba]	[bæ bæ]	*there* [dei]	[babi]
0;11	1;6	[dti]	*byebye* [ba]
bus [bas]	*hi* [hæ]	[de:]	[baba]
put on [baza]	[haj]	0;11	*daddy* [da]
that [za]	1;7	*pretty* [prɪti]	[dada]
1;0	*no* [Oⁿo]	*there* [dɛ:]	[dadi]
down [da]	[no]	*ticktock* [tak]	*dot* [dat]
out [at]	[nu]	1;0	[dati]
away [baˑ'ba]	*hello* [hwow]	*ball* [ba]	*hi* [hai]
pocket [bat]	*squirrel* [gæ]	*Blumen* [bu]	*mommy* [ma]
1;1	[gow]	*da* [da:]	[mami]
fuff [af]	1;8	*opa* [pa]	[mama]
[faf]	*nose* [o]	*papa* [pa-pa]	*no* [no]
put on [bada']	*ear* [iJ]	*piep* [pi]	*see* [si]
1;2	1;9	[pip]	*see that* [siæt]
push [bus]	*boot* [bu]	*pretty* [prti]	*that* [da]
dog [uf]	*nice* [njaj]	*sch-sch* [ʃʃ]	1;4
pie [ba.]	[njajF]	*ticktock* [t'ɪt'a]	*hot* [hat]
1;3	*light* [aj]	[t'at'-t']	*hi* [hai]
duck [dat]	1;10	1;1	[haidi]
lamb [bap]	*car* [gar]	*ball* [ba]	*up* [ap]
1;4	*cheese* [dʒiF]	*bimbam* [bɪ]	[api]
M [am]	*Stevie* [i:v]	*da* [da]	*no* [nodi]
N [an]	*egg* [egɣ]	*Gertrude* [de:da]	[dodi]
in [n]	*apple* [æp]	[dɔ:di]	[noni]
1;5–1;7	*kiss* [giF]	*kick* [ti]	
doll [daˑ]	*up* [ʌf]	*kritze* [tɪtsə]	
S [as]	*mouth* [mæwf]		
O [uˑ]	*eye* [aj]		
R [a]			
nice [nas]			

* When a sound was indeterminate, Menn would use a capital letter, e.g. F means fricative of some kind.

How do these observations capture the facts of acquisition during this period? Table 3 presents the first 25 forms recorded by diary-keeping parents of four normal children. The data come from Velten 1943, Menn 1971, Leopold 1947 and Ingram 1974a. From a glance at these forms we can note several things in regard to the above predictions:

(*a*) With regard to *syllable structure*, CV is common, but VC also occurs. Reduplication occurs, but varies across children. Jennika shows a great deal of it, whereas Joan and Daniel rarely use it. This reflects a general fact that children vary greatly in their use of reduplication. Lastly, each child shows some cases of CVC structures in these forms. Thus it appears that some use of CVC syllables shortly follows in two or three months the appearance of CV and VC syllables. For Jennika, CVC became more frequent than CV at 1;6. Although unsupported by solid research as yet, this suggests that occasional CVC forms appear during the first 50 words, but do not constitute a major part of the child's phonology until after this period.

(*b*) In terms of consonantal segments, those that occur in more than one form for each child are given below:

Joan		Daniel		Hildegard		Jennika	
p	t	b	g	p	t	b	d
b	d	f	h	b	d	t	
f	s		n			s	h
	z						
	ṇ						

When these inventories are combined with those sounds shared by two or more children, the following system occurs:

p	(2)	t	(3)		
b	(4)	d	(3)		
f	(2)	s	(2)	h	(2)

The use of labials agrees with Jakobson's predictions, although the dentals are also prominent and not at all clearly behind. This is despite the fact that the first three children all had labials in their first word. Clearly the velars are not among the first sounds, although Daniel's use of [g] is an exception to this. Ferguson *et al.* (1973) give another example of this and suggest that some children have a preference for velars. The frequency of such cases, however, has yet to be determined. Jakobson's claim about fricatives appearing after homorganic stops is borne out, although it also appears that some fricative sound will occur among the first sounds. This occurs despite the fact that fricatives in general do not constitute a major part of the child's system at this point.

No nasals appear in this group. Individual children did show some use of labials and dental nasals, but overall they were not frequent. Thus it seems that while nasals may occur in important words like *mama* and *no*, they are not obviously among the dominant first sounds of children. With regard to [w] and [h], the latter occurred although the former did not. [w] is apparently an early acquisition, although this data did not show it in the first forms. This may be a reflection of early vocabulary rather than phonological ability, which may also have limited the appearance of some other sounds. It appears that there are overall similarities with a range of individual variations.

(*c*)   Lastly, the vowels showed the following occurrences for each child, again counting only those in at least two forms:

Joan	Daniel		Hildegard	Jennika
u	i	u	i	i
a		o	ɪ, ɛ, ə	a
	æ			
	a		a	
	ai			

Those shared by two or more children are:

i (3)   u (2)

a (4)

Again, once individual variations are eliminated, the occurrences reflect Jakobson's predictions. The basic three-vowel triangle appears, with [a] as the one vowel shared by all four children. Individually, Joan and Jennika show the first split in the vowels, with Joan adding [u], while Jennika adds [i]. Jakobson states that either is possible. Hildegard also has added [i] to [a], but has gone a third step in that several mid lax vowels, [ɪ, ɛ, ə], seem to be used in free variation. This aspect of variation is a common one and will be returned to in the next section. Daniel has the most advanced vowel system. He not only shows the three basic vowels, [i, a, u], but also the onset of others, specifically [o, æ, aj]. Vowels, then, are not acquired during the first 50 words, although at least the basic triangle is probably established in this period.

Another source of information on this period is a recent study by Ferguson and Farwell (1975), who analyse the first 50 words of three normal children. They note that Jakobson discusses the phonology of children during this period as unaffected by the words in which the sounds appear. They argue strongly that one needs to consider the *role of individual lexical items* in phonological acquisition. That is, the child is not simply acquiring a system of sounds, but also a set of lexical items. The acquisition of specific patterns and sounds may be greatly influenced by the words in which they occur.

They demonstrate this by pointing out three specific characteristics of acquisition during this period. The first of these has to do with the occurrence of *variation* in the production of words. Children do not simply acquire a sound and produce it correctly, but rather show alternations in its use. While this variation may be in some cases across lexical items, there are at least two ways that it is affected by specific lexical items. The first is by a phenomenon referred to as 'trade-off', a process first observed by Edwards and Garnica (1973). The latter noted that the acquisition of a new part of a word may distort the production of another part. For example, the acquisition of a final consonant may affect the occurrence of an initial one. Secondly, Ferguson and Farwell note that variation seems to vary across lexical items. For example, some items may be quite stable, and be pronounced the same for several months. Others, however, may be quite variable. A complete picture of variation, then, cannot be achieved without the examination of specific lexical items.

They also use this process to raise serious questions about Jakobson's claim that the young child has a set of phonological contrasts, and consequently a system that functions rather like an adult's. This refers to the ability to use sounds to distinguish different words. A child who has a phonological contrast between two sounds such as [b] and [d] for example, can be said to use them to keep words distinct, such as [ba] versus [da], where each has its own meaning. Ferguson and Farwell give an example with [m] and [n] from a child in their study. The child had some words with [m], some with [m] varying with [n], and a few with [n]. It appears that the child does not yet have a clear [m], [n] contrast. Rather, it is gradually developing, and only exists between certain words. They use this observation to conclude, 'It does seem from our data that it is often impossible to make well-motivated claims about phonological contrasts in the usual sense at these early stages, as some might wish to do' (17).

Another kind of evidence for this conclusion can be found in Braine 1971. At one early point in his development, Braine's son had the following total vocabulary:

see	[diː]
that or *there*	[da] [dʌ]
juice	[duː]
no	[do]
hi	[ʔai]

Here, one could possibly speak of an initial contrast in the child's speech between [d] and zero, i.e. no consonant at all, as in [ʔai] for *hi*. To test this, Braine taught the child a word [iː], which was to mean *eat* or *food*. It was used by Braine in relation to meals. The child learned the word, but pronounced it as [diː]. Next, Braine taught the child the invented word [dai] to contrast with [hai] for *hi*. The child learned it, but pronounced it as [da] or [dʌ]. Braine concludes that the child's initial [d] did not have contrastive (or phonemic) status.

This finding that the child may not yet have a viable system of contrastive sounds is in keeping with the child's cognitive stage at this point. Recall that the child between 1;0 and 1;6 is still in Piaget's sensori-motor period. That is, the child still does not have the representational ability to acquire language, which for Piaget begins about 1;6. What the child has now is an image of the sounds for words, but these images are still unstable. This is because the child still needs to coordinate the attachment of this verbal image to the entity in the world to which it refers. It is because of this that words during this time are so frequently generalized, and used to refer to a wide variety of things, with a link that is not always clear. Later the child learns that words are social signs, with an accepted reference. He learns to coordinate the relation between a set of sounds and their referent. This occurs after 1;6, and it may well be that the development of contrastive ability likewise does not appear until after that time.

A second observation of Ferguson and Farwell concerns the pronunciation of words during this stage. It sometimes happens that the child's pronunciation of a word is better, in the sense of more adult-like, at first than it is later on. That is, the child will pronounce a word fairly well, and then show progressively reduced pronunciations over the months. These could be called *advanced forms*, in that they show pronunciation beyond that expected for the child's level of development. They also have the characteristic of becoming less advanced as they become part of the child's system. The most famous example is taken from Leopold's daughter Hildegard for her pronunciation of *pretty*. Its production over several months is shown below:

pretty	0;10	[prəti]
	0;11	[prɪti]
	1;0	[pɾtɪ]
	1;1	[prɪti] [prəti]
	1;3	[pʃɪti]
	1;4	[pwɪti] [pəti] [pyɪti]
	1;9	[pɪti]
	1;10	[bɪdi]

There are points worth making in regard to these phenomena. Their nature and occurrence has yet to be studied. For example, it is not clear just how frequent they are, nor whether or not they are restricted to this period of acquisition. Even though they may be frequent, Hildegard's example is one of the few well-documented cases. If these phenomena only occur in this period, it is consistent with the position that the child is not yet using a productive phonological system. During the next stage the child will use a number of simplifying processes. One of these is *voicing*, where stops are voiced before vowels. Note that Hildegard's form of *pretty* finally becomes [bɪdi], undergoing this process. If these phenomena occur in other periods, it suggests that words are first acquired outside the child's system, and only later enter into it. Further research will need to answer questions of this sort.

A last characteristic of acquisition during the first 50 words concerns the child's selection of words. Ferguson and Farwell show that the child shows preferences for the kinds of words acquired. For example, one of the children they studied acquired words with labial stops only if they were [b]. No words beginning with [p] were acquired for several sessions. Likewise Hildegard preferred [b] words until around 1;10 or 1;11 when several [p] words were acquired. Thus it appears that children are highly selective in the sound pattern of words they acquire.

These, then, are some general aspects of the earliest stage of phonological development. The child's vocabulary is small and grows slowly. The child's phonetic inventory is small, with some basic segments as well as individual variations. The word appears to play an important role in acquisition here, and contrasts seem to occur more between words than sound classes. The child does not seem to have a productive sound system, a development that becomes the major part of the next stage of acquisition, when the child begins the active process of acquisition of a complex set of linguistic rules.

2.33   The phonology of the simple morpheme

About the middle of the second year, two steps occur in the linguistic development of the child. There is a sudden, rapid growth of vocabulary and the onset of two-word utterances. At this point, rapid phonological development also begins. In terms of syntax, several stages have been suggested as occurring between 1;6 and 4;0. Brown (1973) discusses these in terms of mean length of utterance (i.e. mean number of morphemes per utterance), and labels his stages I to V. In the first stage, from 1;6 to 2;0 approximately, there is the growth of multiple word utterances with one-word utterances still being the most frequent. By stage V, complex sentences begin to appear, and the child has mastered a great deal of syntax. These and other stages, e.g. those of Nice (1925), are discussed in Ingram (in press). There are probably phonological developments that accompany each of these stages. The specific facts, however, await research. As a result, this discussion will treat this general cognitive stage without breaking it down into substages. Basically, it is the period in which the child develops his or her perceptual abilities, acquires a broad inventory of phonetic elements, loses a variety of simplifying phonological processes and acquires a phonological system of contrasts.

2.331   The development of perception

There was little mentioned about perception during the last section on development between 1;0 and 1;6. With the onset of the development of a system of phonemic contrasts in speech production, it can be assumed that similar progress occurs in the child's perception. That is, the child develops the ability to determine which speech sounds are used to signal differences in meaning.

Shvachkin (1973) has made the most extensive study of children's ability to hear phonemic distinctions. He was interested in following the development of this ability in very young children between one and two years of age. To do this, he established the following approach. He taught each child a name for each of three different objects, e.g. *bak*, *mak*, *zub*. This was done one object at a time. Then, he placed all three before the child and requested one, e.g. *bak* versus *mak*. If the child heard the difference between [b] and [m] he would hand the correct object over. In this way Shvachkin proceeded through various contrasts, testing the child's ability to hear them. The subjects were 19 Russian children who were·0;10 to 1;6 at the beginning of the study. Each was tested longitudinally for periods ranging from 4 to 8 months.

The first finding was that the development of phonemic perception was gradual over this time, beginning with general contrasts at about 1;0 to more elaborate ones by 2;0. More specifically, he found 12 stages of phonemic perception. These are summarized in table 4. They can be broken down into two periods—vowel

Table 4   Shvachkin's stages of phonemic perception

	Stage-distinction	Substages	Examples
1	Vowels	1	a v. other vowels
		2	i–u; e–o; i–o; e–u
		3	i–e; e–u
2	Presence v. absence of consonant		bok–ok; vek–ek; d'ik–ik
3	Sonorants v. stops		m–b; r–d; n–g
4	Palatalized v. non-palatalized consonants		n–n'; m–m'; b–b'; d–d'; v–v'; z–z'; l–l'; r–r'
5	Between sonorants	1	nasals v. liquids m–l; m–r, n–l; n–r; n–y; m–y
		2	m–n
		3	l–r
6	Sonorants v. continuants		m–z; l–x; n–ž
7	Labials v. linguals		b–d; b–g; v–z; f–x
8	Stops v. spirants		b–v; d–ž; k–x; d–ž
9	Pre- v. post-linguals		d–g; s–x; š–x
10	Voiced v. voiceless consonants		p–b; t–d; k–g; f–v; š–ž; s–z
11	Between sibilants		ž–z; š–s
12	Liquids v. /y/		r–y; l–y

distinctions (stage 1) and consonant distinctions (stages 2–12). Also, Shvachkin suggests six levels:

(1) Distinction of vowels—stage 1
(2) Distinction of presence of consonants—stage 2
(3) Distinction of sonorants and voiced stops—stage 3
(4) Distinction of palatalized and nonpalatalized consonants—stage 4
(5) Distinction of sonorants—stages 5, 6
(6) Distinction of obstruents—stages 7, 8, 9, 10, 11, 12.

Although observed in Russian children, these stages may be taken as possible general stages of development for children learning other languages. Except for stage 4, which refers to a sound distinction not present in English, these can be carried over to English. In fact, a recent replication of this study has been done in English by Garnica (1973), who has refined some of the methodological problems of the Russian study. She tested 16 children between the ages of 1;5 and 1;10, and found, like Shvachkin, that children had not yet developed the ability to distinguish phonemic perception. She also found that similar stages occurred, but not with as much consistency as expected. Garnica attributes this to more variability between stages than allowed by the original formulation. In general, children are still developing perceptual ability between one and two years of age.

At first glance, one might find such results contradictory to those of researchers who have shown infants to have good perceptual ability. It is necessary, however, to separate linguistic and nonlinguistic (or phonemic v. phonetic) perception. The studies with infants are dealing with nonlinguistic perception; the child needs only to hear a difference between two sounds. In linguistic studies the sounds are labels of objects, i.e. they are words. This new aspect of meaning introduces a new problem into perception. This is much like a *décalage* in the sense that Piaget has used the term, i.e. an ability developed on one cognitive level has to be relearned at the next level.

These results do not suggest that perception is complete by 2;0. Both these studies only tested CVC syllables. It is possible that more complex syllables introduce perceptual difficulties so that the growth of perception may continue to develop over the years. Edwards (1974) has also tested perception by using the Shvachkin approach as developed by Garnica. While still using CVC syllables, she focused on the differences between fricative pairs, specifically: [s]–[z]; [f]–[v]; [š]–[ž]; and [θ]–[ð]. She tested 28 children between 1;8 and 3;11 and found that '(a) children as late as three do not have complete phonemic perception, (b) phonemic perception develops gradually, generally in advance of production, and (c) the order of acquisition shows trends toward uniformity but is not universal' (67).

This fact, that perception may not be complete at age 1;0 and may develop gradually over several years, is not one that has been appreciated in much of the child language literature. Rather, it is more common to find suggestions that perception is complete at an early age (e.g. Smith 1973). This may be because children occasionally demonstrate their advanced perception. For example, Jespersen (1964) cites an example of a French girl who said *tosson* for both *garçon* (boy and *cochon* (pig), but protested when others misused her term. Berko and Brown (1960) cite an example from a boy, Adam, who protested when the adult said Adam's form of [fɪs] referring to a *fish*. Adam protested 'not fis, fis!' Smith (1973) has cited examples of this kind from his son (A). When Smith tried to get A to say *ship*, which A pronounced as [sɪp], A was aware of this and said, 'No, I can only say [sɪp]' (137). All these, however, simply show that perception precedes production. They do not demonstrate that it is complete.

2.332 Perception and production

If perception is not complete, the question arises of the relationship between perception and production. Shvachkin (1973) concluded that there is a definite interaction between the two. He states 'a child who has mastered certain sounds can discriminate them faster than a child who has not mastered the same sounds' (113). This suggests a close relationship, where productive skills facilitate perceptive ones. Conversely, he suggests that sounds that are not produced by the child are discriminated later.

Others have taken the opposite position. Both Peizer and Olmsted (1969) and Salus and Salus (1974) have suggested that sounds are not pronounced correctly until they are perceived. Consequently, sounds that are not pronounced later are also sounds that are perceived late. In this approach it is perception that facilitates production rather than the reverse.

The above studies on perception have all arrived at the finding of incomplete perception through direct testing of perceptual contrasts. Waterson (1971), on the other hand, has also been able to demonstrate this from a child's productive speech. In fact, she uses the argument of incomplete perception to explain children's words which do not at first glance look like reductions of adult models. The child she has observed, P, was approximately 1;6 at the time, with a vocabulary of about 155 words. He was then just beginning to acquire a phonology of simple morphemes. Waterson argues that the child at this time does not perceive the entire segmental structure of the adult world. Instead, 'a child perceives only certain of the features of the adult utterance and reproduces only those that he is able to cope with' (181). The child establishes general perceptual types, which are structures into which words fall. For example, a child may prefer words with nasality, and establish a structure which incorporates words with nasals. Waterson's examples from P of five types are given in table 5.

Table 5   Five structural types, adapted from Waterson 1971, with examples of each

Type	Structure	Examples
I	Labial structure wV(wV)	*fly* [wæ] [bβæ] 1;5 [βæ] [væ] [bβæ] 1;6 *barrow* [wæwæ] 1;5 [bʌwu] 1;6 *flower* [væ] [væwæ] 1;6
II	Continuant structure VhV	*Rooney* [ẽh̃ẽ/h̃ẽh̃ẽ] 1;6 *honey* [aɦu:] 1;8 *hymn, angel* [aɦɔ] [æhə] [ãh̃ʊ̃]
III	Sibilant structure (C)Vš	*fish* [ɪʃ] [ʊʃ] 1;6 *fetch* [ɪʃ] 1;6 *vest* [ʊʃ] 1;6 *brush* [byʃ] 1;6 *dish* [dɪʃ] 1;6
IV	Stop structure CVCV	*biscuit* [be:be:] 1;6 *Bobby* [bæbu:] 1;6 *pudding* [pupu] 1;6 *bucket* [bæbu:] 1;6 *kitty* [tɪti] 1;6 *dirty* [dɟ:ti] 1;6
V	Nasal structure ɲVɲV	*finger* [ɲẽ:ɲẽ] [ɲi:ɲɪ] *window* [ɲe:ɲe] *another* [ɲaɲa] *Randall* [ɲaɲø̰]

According to Waterson's analysis, P has five basic perceptual structures. The labial structure is one that is CV or CVCV where the C is a labial sound, usually [w]. The continuant structure is VCV with C being a glottal fricative. The sibilant structure is (C)V[š]; a word that does not have an [š], such as *vest* gets incorporated. The stop structure is CV CV, where the stops are usually the same. Lastly, the nasal structure is one of [ɲ]V[ɲ]V. Words which are marked by nasality are then placed in this structure.

These types show the kinds of preferences already mentioned by Ferguson and Farwell. That is, it shows that the child is a selective listener. While groupings like this are probably most abundant in the earliest stages of development, they show the interrelation between perception and production, and the need to consider the child to be doing more than simply substituting one sound for another.

2.333 The phonetic inventory

With the above caution in mind, we can now observe how the child's phonetic ability improves between the ages of 1;6 and 4;0. As we have seen, at the start the child has a very reduced syllable structure, with a small set of basic sounds. By 4;0, however, this has been broadened greatly.

Two studies in particular have presented information on the ages of acquisition of English speech sounds, those of Templin (1957) and Olmsted (1971). An examination of each of these provides a survey of the acquisition of English sounds.

Templin gave an articulation test to 480 children, 60 (balanced for sex) at each of the following ages (within one month)—3;0, 3;6, 4;0, 4;6, 5;0, 6;0, 7;0, 8;0. The test consisted of words that measured 176 sounds—69 single consonants, 90 consonant clusters (or blends), 12 vowels and 5 diphthongs. The words were elicited from the children through either spontaneous naming of a picture or imitation of the word as spoken by the experimenter. The responses were transcribed on the scene by Templin without the use of a tape recorder. A sound was considered acquired if 75 per cent of the children at an age level pronounced it correctly.

Overall, initial position was the easiest one for consonants, followed by medial position and then final position. The differences between each was significant. In regard to specific sounds, table 6 shows those segments (and their positions in words

Table 6   Sounds acquired and not acquired by age 4;0, based on Templin 1957*

Class	Acquired by 4;0	Not acquired (Age acquired)
Stops	p(3) t–, –t k(4) b(4) d(4) g(4)	–t–(6)
Affricates	ǰ–	č (4;6) –ǰ–(5) –ǰ(7)
Fricatives	f(3) s–, –s–, š–, –š –v– –z–	θ(6) ð–(6) –ð–(7) –ð(7) v–(6) –v(6) z–(7) –z(7) ž(7) –s(4;6)
Nasals	m(3) n(3) ŋ(3)	
Glides	w(3) y(3;6)	
Liquids	l–, –l–, r(4)	–l(6)
Vowels	all acquired (3)	

* A dash indicates position in a word. p–, for example, refers to initial p. If no dashes are given, then all positions are referred to.

if different) that are acquired by age 4;0, and those that are not. First, all vowels are acquired by 3;0. This precedence of vowel acquisition parallels that found in the perception studies. *Vowels are acquired before consonants.* Next, all the nasals are acquired; these are followed by glides. Stops are also nearly all acquired, with the exception of [–t–], a sound of questionable status because of its flapping in many English dialects. The sounds that show predominant incomplete acquisition are the fricatives and affricates. These require several more years for complete acquisition.

While single consonants show major gains, the clusters are not so widely acquired. Table 7 shows the acquisition of these over the groups observed. Certain trends can be noted from these results. For one, [s] + Nasal or Stop clusters appear to be acquired initially. This is also the case for stop + liquid clusters. There is a

Table 7 Consonant clusters acquired, and not acquired by 4;0, with ages provided, based on Templin 1957

Cluster	Acquired by 4;0	Not acquired
Initial		
s + nasal	sm–(4), sn–(4)	
s + stop	sp–(4), st–(4), sk–(4)	
s + L/G*		sl–(7); sw–(7)
s + stop + L/G		str–(5), skr–(7), spl–(7), spr–(7) skw–(6)
Stop + liquid	pl–(4) pr–(4), tr–(4), kl–(4), gl–(4), kr–(4), bl–(4), br–(4), dr–(4)	gr–(4;6)
Stop + glide	tw–(4), kw–(4)	
Fricative + L/G		fr–(4;5), fl–(5), θr–(7), šr–(7), sl–(7), sw–(7)
Final		
s + stop		–sk(7), –st(7), –sp(8)
Liquid + Stop	–lp(4), –lt(4)	–rp(4;6), –lb(4;6), –lk(6), –rb(6), –rg(6)
Liquid + Fricative		–lf(4;6), –rf(4;6), –rθ(6), –rj(6), –lz(7), –lθ(7)
Liquid + nasal	–rm(3;6)	
Nasal + Obstr.	–ŋk(3), –mp(3;6)	–nt(6), –nd(6), –nθ(6)
Nasal + C + C	–mpt(4), –mps(4)	
Stop + obstr.	–pt(3;6), –ks(3;6)	–kt(8)
Stop + C + C		–kst(7)
Fricative + Obstr.	–ft(4)	–jd(7)

* L/G indicates Liquid or Glide.

trend for final nasal + stop acquisition, but this is not widely tested. Triple clusters are generally not acquired in either position. Also, fricative + liquids are not acquired initially, and liquid + obstruent clusters are not acquired. In summary, the clusters that have been acquired by 4;0 are:

Word initial	Word final
/s/ + Nasal	Nasal + Stop
Liquid	
Stop	
Stop + Liquid	

The rest are acquired in the following stage.

(There is further discussion of the acquisition of clusters in section 2.334 on phonological processes.)

In using Templin's results, several cautions need to be kept in mind. There was only one word per sound per child. Also, the mode of elicitation was either spontaneous or imitated. Both of these factors could make a difference in the age of acquisition. Templin argues that her study in 1947 demonstrated that neither of these makes a difference. However, neither of these issues has been resolved to date. It is not clear whether the word in which a sound appears makes a difference to its articulation. Also, as will be discussed, the acquisition of a sound is gradual. That is, the child progressively varies between correct and incorrect pronunciation. Giving one word, however, assumes incorrectly that acquisition is all or nothing. Lastly, there are suggestions that imitation leads to better pronunciation (Olmsted 1971). All these methodological questions will be discussed in greater detail in chapter 4.

Another caution to be kept in mind is that general guidelines ignore the question of *individual variation*. Children will vary greatly from one another with regard to their acquisition of the different sounds in question. Sander (1961) was concerned with this dilemma in determining a fixed date for the acquisition of a sound. To overcome this, he suggested giving age ranges of acquisition, from the point at which a reasonable number of children begin to acquire a sound to a point when most have it. Using data from Wellman *et al.* (1931) and Templin, he determined age ranges of acquisition of English consonants. For any consonant, the range starts from the median age of customary articulation until the age where 90 per cent of all children are customarily producing it. Table 8 summarizes his results. Thus children may differ by as much as 3 years in attaining correct pronunciation of specific English sounds.

Table 8   Average age estimates for the acquisition of English sounds, based on Sander 1961

Sounds	Median age of customary usage	Age of 90% of subjects
p, m, h, n, w	1;6	3;0
b	1;6	4;0
k, g, d	2;0	4;0
t, ŋ	2;0	6;0
f, y	2;6	4;0
r, l	3;0	6;0
s	3;0	8;0
č, š	3;6	7;0
z	4;0	7;0
j	4;0	7;0
v	4;0	8;0
θ	4;6	7;0
ð	5;0	8;0
ž	6;0	8;6

Another problem of Templin's study is that it ignores the fact that all English sounds are not of equal frequency. By eliciting all sounds once, this is assumed. Olmsted (1971) avoided this by determining acquisition of sounds based on spontaneous speech sounds of children. His subjects were 100 children ranging from 1;3 to 4;6 years of age. Spontaneous speech samples of various length were collected from each child. Olmsted examined a variety of aspects of acquisition, including frequency of individual sounds, the susceptibility of sounds to error, substitutions, variation in pronunciation etc. Generally, he found that the most common errors were of place, followed by friction, voicing and nasality. Within place, labials were pronounced best, followed by equal scores for alveolars and velars. By far the worst places were interdental and post alveolar positions.

Olmsted also looked at the order of acquisition. He defined a sound as acquired as follows: a sound is acquired if more subjects in an age group attempted and correctly pronounced a sound 50 per cent more than subjects that did not. His age groups were, with number of subjects: 1;3–1;11 (17), 2;0–2;5 (32), 2;6–2;11 (25), 3;0–3;5 (13), 3;6–3;11 (7), 4;0–4;6 (6). Based on this measure, table 9 shows sounds that are and are not acquired by age 4;0. When compared with Templin's findings in table 6, a remarkable similarity occurs. Despite very different kinds of data and measures of acquisition, both show very similar results concerning the sounds acquired over this period.

Table 9 Sounds acquired and not acquired by age 4;0 in Olmsted 1971. If no position is marked, all positions are referred to.

Class	Acquired by 4;0			Not acquired		
Stops	p	t–, –t	k	t–		
	b	d	g			
Affricates		–č		č–	–č–	
		–ǰ–		ǰ–	–ǰ	
Fricatives	f –θ–, –θ	s	š	ð–	–ð–	ð–
	v	–z–, –z		z–	–ž–	–z
				θ–		
Nasals	m	n		ŋ		
Glides	w		y			
Liquids		l–	r	–l–,	–l	
Vowels	all acquired					

Before leaving Olmsted's study, one last point should be mentioned. Olmsted emphasizes correctly that previous studies erred in considering acquisition as an all or nothing matter. Throughout his study, individual subjects continually varied in success and error with the sounds attempted. Therefore, *children do not acquire individual sounds suddenly, but gradually over time*, with extended periods where the sound is both correctly and incorrectly produced.

2.334 Phonological processes

When discussing the acquisition of individual sounds, the impression is given that acquisition is concerned with sounds in isolation from each other. In fact, the opposite is often the case. During this period of 1;6 to 4;0 when many words are incorrectly pronounced, there are several very general simplifying processes that affect entire classes of sounds. Here I shall briefly present the most general of these processes.

Syllable structure processes One category of processes operates to simplify the structure of syllables. This is accomplished in various ways. The general tendency is to reduce all words to a basic CV syllable. This may be done by the deletion of final consonants, the reduction of clusters to one segment, and the deletion of unstressed syllables. Reduplication can also be viewed as a syllable structure process in that it simplifies the production of a second syllable by repeating the first.

Deletion of final consonants Table 3 with the first 25 words of 4 children reveals that there is an initial tendency for children to delete final consonants, especially in CVC syllables. This appears to be a common process in the early months of this period. Little is actually known about how this process gradually disappears. Irwin (1951) reports a marked increase in the use of final consonants by age 3;0. In Templin, less than 10 per cent of the final consonants were deleted at age 3. So, the process appears to disappear about that age.

With regard to the manner in which it is deleted, Renfrew (1966) has proposed ten stages in the development of final consonants in children with a persistent deletion of final consonants. Although proposed for deviant children, they can be used to compare with normal children. The stages are summarized in table 10. At least one of the stages appears to be similar to normal development. This is the early appearance of nasals in final position.

Table 10   Stages in the appearance of final consonants for some deviant children, based on Renfrew 1966

Stage	Pattern
1, 2, 3	No final consonants. In Stage 3, CVCs are imitated with final vowel, e.g. *dog* [dɔ–gə]
4	Appearance of final nasals: [m] correct, [n], [ŋ] vary
5	Nasals are correct; [l] appears finally
6	[ʔ] is used for all stops finally
7	[p], [b], [d] are used finally, still replace [t], [k], [g]—in latter, vowel is lengthened to indicate deleted stop
8	Final [t] is now used. Some attempts at fricatives
9	All final consonants, including fricatives, are correct, except [k], [g]
10	Articulation normal

Ingram (1974b) proposes two specific hypotheses about the development of final consonants. The study notes a general tendency for the early use of velar consonants in final position. The strong hypothesis is that velars are acquired before other consonants in final position. While this is too strong to apply to all children, there do appear to be cases for which this is true. The weak hypothesis is that children acquire velars in final position before initial position. Again, this is still unsupported although there are individual cases showing it.

In summary, final consonant deletion as a simplifying process by and large is lost between 1;6 and 3;0. The order of appearance of final consonants is not clear, but it appears that use of vowel length, glottal stop and nasals may all be involved in the earliest stages. There is also the possibility that final position may be easier than initial position for the appearance of some sounds.

Deletion of unstressed syllables   This is a common process during the early part of this period. At first, as already mentioned, the child's words are primarily monosyllables (or reduplication of the basic syllable, cf. below). As a result, some part of adult words with more than one syllable is lost. The part that is lost is the unstressed syllable. The following stages can be suggested, although they are by and large impressionistic.

Table 11   Impressionistic stages in the development of stressed syllables with hypothetical examples.*

	Bisyllabic words			Trisyllabic words			
Stress pattern	Ś S		S Ś	Ś S S		S Ś S	
Example	apple		behind	telephone		potato	
Stage 1	æp		aind	(none)		(none)	
Stage 2	æpl		aind	tɛfon		teto	
Stage 3	æpl		aind	tɛləfon		teto	
Stage 4	æpl		bəhaind	tɛləfon		teto	
Stage 5	æpl		bəhaind	tɛləfon		pəteto	

* For simplicity, correct segmental productions are given although presumably there would also be errors in them.

In the first stage, only monosyllables appear. Adult words with three syllables usually are not even attempted at this time. Real examples can be found in table 3: Joan *pocket* [bat] 1;0, Daniel *apple* [æp] 1;10, Hildegard *Blumen* [bu] 1;0, Jennika *blanket* [ba] 1;3. This stage probably is typical of the Phonology of the First 50 Words. In the second stage, two syllable productions appear, and two deletion processes occur. First, initial unstressed syllables are reduced; second, all unstressed syllables in three syllable words are dropped. In the third stage, the deletion of unstressed initial syllables continues, but medial syllables now occur. This stage occurred in A (Smith 1973) at the age of 2;2 to 2;3, with the following examples:

Robbie	[wɔbiː]	*away*	[weː]	*telephone*	[dɛwiːbuːn]
tomato	['maːdo]				

At this point deletion of unstressed syllables has been limited to initial ones.

In the proposed fourth stage, initial unstressed syllables are attempted in bisyllabic words, but not as much as in trisyllabic ones. The following two words from Smith 1973 exemplify this for his son A:

away	[weː]	[wei]	2;2	*banana*	[baːnə]	2;2
	[ə'weː]	[weː]	2;3		[baːnə]	2;8
	[ə'wei]		2;4		[bə'naːnə]	3;1

This development, however, needs to be considered with caution. Smith points out that 'there was considerable inconsistency in A's treatment of words with an unstressed initial syllable' (172). This variation no doubt results from the generally gradual process of acquisition. That Smith does not show an appreciation of this inherent variation has already been pointed out by Olmsted (1974).

At the onset of stage 4, there may be a period when the child attempts unstressed syllables by a single phonetic shape. Smith points out that his son, during the period from 3;6 to 3;11, used the shape *ri* for many initial unstressed syllables, e.g. *attack* [riː'tæk]; *arrange* [ri'reinz]; *disturb* [ris'təːv]; *elastic* [riː'æstik] etc. (172). For a short period, *in-* was tried instead. Stage 5 marks the appropriate adult pronunciation.

This process lasts longer than that of the deletion of final consonants. It appears to affect syllables in some way at least up to age 4 and beyond.

Reduplication The process of reduplication is one in which the child repeats the syllable of the word. Examples from table 3 include: Joan *away* [ba'ba], Daniel *bye bye* [baba], Hildegard *Papa* [papa], Jennika *daddy* [dada]. Besides these total reduplications, it is common to find in English partial reduplications ending with *i*, e.g. Jennika's *blanket* [babi], *daddy* [dadi], *mommy* [mami]. Jennika showed productive use of this in forms such as *hi* [haidi], *up* [api], and *no* [nodi], all taken from table 3. Other examples can be found in Ross 1937 and Hamp 1974; the rule is discussed with further examples in Ingram 1974a.

Two aspects of reduplication are worth noting. First, it appears to be an early process of acquisition, most common in the phonology of the first 50 Words. Secondly, children do vary in their use of it. As noted, Jennika was an active reduplicater, while others are much less so. It may also have some relation to the child's ability to produce final consonants. If a child has difficulty, the use of some partial reduplication can assist in this, e.g. *dog* [da] or [daga]. Attempts to study the interrelation between the two processes, however, have not been made.

The reduction of clusters Like the deletion of unstressed syllables, this process is one that has several stages and lasts in some form for a long time before finally being lost. It is the process by which the child simplifies clusters of consonants, usually by deleting one of them. These deletions in most cases are nct random, but show predictable patterns. As mentioned in an earlier section, clusters develop in different sequences of acquisition (cf. table 7). Data like this show the points of acquisition of the clusters, but not the stages that occur between the first attempts at clusters and final correct production.

There are general stages that apply across all the types. These are adopted from Greenlee 1974 and may be stated as follows, with examples of how *play* would be pronounced at each:

Stage 1   Deletion of entire cluster [ey]
Stage 2   Reduction of cluster to one member [pey]
Stage 3   Use of cluster with substitution for one of the members [pwey]
Stage 4   Correct articulation [pley].

Greenlee has demonstrated the generality of these as well as other patterns shown in the acquisition of clusters.

The first stage, the deletion of the entire cluster would be early in development, and affected by the deletion of final consonants for final clusters. Since most clusters are reduced to one member in the early months (i.e. stage 2), it is not clear that stage 1 is a widespread or even common step. The only examples that Greenlee gives are from two French children; Edmond 'wheelbarrow' *brouette* 'ouette' at 2;0 (19), 'pencil' *crayon* 'iyon' 2;0 (19), and Louis 'grey' *gris* [i] 2;0, and 'big' *grand* [arã] 2;4.

The reduction of the cluster to one member is common and widespread, and lasts for several months. Olmsted (1971, 212) shows that this was the most common treatment of clusters by his subjects. The member that is deleted is often predictable; the most common process is the *deletion of the marked member*. Those that are fairly well attested are given below:

Deletion of marked member of a cluster (Examples from A, in Smith 1973)

Type

I   /s/ + Consonant Delete /s/

	initial			final	
stop	[tʰɔp]	(2;8)	desk	[dɛk]	(2;8)
small	[mɔ:]	(2;4)			
slide	[laid]	(2;7)			

II   Stop + Liquid Delete liquid

	initial			final (order reversed)	
clock	[ɟɔk]	(2;2)	milk	[mik]	(2;2)
bring	[ḅiŋ]	(2;5)			

III   Fricative + Liquid/Glide Delete liquid/glide

	initial	
from	[fɔm]	(2;10)

IV   Nasal and Obstruent

Stage 1 Delete nasal	Stage 2 Delete stop if voiced
bump [bʌp] (2;2)	*round* [daun] (2;2)
tent [dɛt] (2;2)	*mend* [mɛn] (2;2)

The two stages given with type IV represents the fact that while the nasal tends to be deleted, when the stop is voiced, it may eventually become subject to deletion.

While the deletion of the marked members is by far the more common, occasionally children will show *deletion of the unmarked member*. Unlike the former, however, this appears to be less frequent and to occur for a briefer period. Smith's son A had the following examples of this:

I   *stop*   [sɔp]   (3;0) with deletion of [t] instead of [s];
II   *trolley*   [lɔliː]   (2;2) with deletion of [t] instead of [r];
III   *three*   [liː]   (2;5).

It has yet to be determined if and when children choose this alternative.

Another process that occurs in stage 2 and continues into stage 3 is that of the weakening of stops. This is actually an assimilation process but is discussed here because of its close relation with cluster reduction processes. Observe my own daughter's forms for the production of adult *truck*:

[gʌk] 1;9	[fʌk] 2;0
[gʌk] 1;10	[frʌk] 2;0
[kʌk] 1;10	

With the onset of a liquid of some kind, the stop weakens, most frequently to the fricative [f]. Since the first appearance of a segment for the liquid is most often the glide [w], this may be an assimilation to the labiality of this element, as well as the loss of closure. Below are some further examples taken from Greenlee 1973, from a boy named Buddy between 2;3 and 2;4. Notice the onset of stage 3, and the occurrence of the assimilation with fricatives.

tree [fwij]	*three* [fwij]
truck [fʌk]	*sweet* [fwij]
twins [fwins]	*throw* [fow]

Since acquisition is gradual, the process will occur both with and without deletion. Greenlee shows this with other examples from Buddy at 3;0: *slow* [fwow] ~ [fow]; *throw* [fow] ~ [fwow]; *flew* [fwuw] ~ [fuw].

With stage 3, clusters begin, but they are still not correct by adult standards. Most frequently, there is a substitution of some kind for one of the members. At this point, it is important to emphasize that the reduction of clusters to one member will still take place. The appearance of stage 3 for any type of cluster represents the continuation of former simplifications plus the first appearances of combinations. A diversity of the kinds of substitutions that may occur are given in Olmsted 1971. Greenlee (1974) provides some of the most common, which are exemplified below:

r → l	*bread* [blɛd]	A (2;7)
r → w	*brown* [bʷaun]	A (2;6)
l → w	*sleep* [fwijp]	Buddy (3;0)

There are two less common processes that also occasionally appear at this stage. They both deal with clusters in a similar fashion, by separating them in some way to keep a basic CVC syllable structure. The first of these is the insertion of a vowel (or epenthesis). Examples are from A: *bread* [bərɛd] (2;6), *play* [bəlei] (2;6). Olmsted (1971) points out also that this is a relatively infrequent process. The second process is the migration of one of the members. In this case the cluster is reduced by moving one of the members away. An example from A is *blue* pronounced [buːl] at 2;6. Both of these are infrequent but available processes. All of the various processes will vary during the latter part of stage 3 with correct articulation. Greenlee (1974, (92) gives these examples from A showing this:

bread   2;6   (23)   [b̥ɛd] ~ [b̥rɛd] ~ [b̥lɛd]
          2;7   (17)   [blɛd]   [brɛd].

Stage 4 is reached for any cluster when correct production dominates, say 90 per cent.

It is important to remember that these stages and processes refer to individual cluster types. One which is acquired early will have gone through all these when one which is being acquired may be only at stage 2. These, then, are different from stages of appearance which would be based on table 7. Below the stages and processes are summarized:

Stage 1	*Stage 2*	*Stage 3*
Deletion of cluster	Deletion of marked member (Deletion of unmarked member) (Weakening of stop) (Labial assimilation)	Substitution of member (Labial assimilation) (Insertion of vowel) (Migration of member)
Examples with *truck*		
[ʌk]	[tʌk] ([rʌk]) ([sʌk]) ([fʌk])	[twʌk] ([fwʌk]) ([tərʌk]) ([tʌrk])

Assimilatory processes   If one takes a strict substitutional approach to acquisition, there will always be some unusual replacements for segments. These will be the result of assimilation patterns that occur in children's speech. Assimilation is the process in which a sound becomes similar to (or is influenced by) another sound in the word. Examination of any child's speech will provide examples of these. Unfortunately, little is actually known about the range, limits and potentialities of assimilating processes in children's speech. An exception is the valuable discussion in Leopold (1947, (207–12). Here I will provide a survey of some of the kinds that have been observed to date.

Assimilation can be either *contiguous* or *noncontiguous*. By contiguous is meant that the element causing the assimilation is next to the affected element. Also, the assimilation can be *progressive* or *regressive*. Assimilation is regressive if the affected segment precedes the one that influences it. It is progressive if the affected segment follows. With these distinctions, there are at least four aspects of child speech that can be discussed—CC, CV or VC, CVC and VCV shapes. These are: (*1*) contiguous assimilation between consonants, (*2*) contiguous assimilation between a consonant and a vowel, (*3*) noncontiguous assimilation between consonants, and (*4*) noncontiguous assimilation between vowels.

(*1*)   In regard to contiguous assimilation between consonants, one example has already been discussed. This is the process of the weakening of stops and labial assimilation in clusters. This appears to be one of the more common cases of this kind of assimilation.

A related process to this is the process that devoices word final consonants. This can be said to be assimilatory in that the stop assimilates to the silence. There is a tendency for children to unvoice consonants when they appear at the end of a word. Some examples from Velten are *knob* [nap] (1;10), *mud* [mat] (1;9), *egg* [ut] (1;9), *hose* [hus] (1;9). This process, of course, depends on the disappearance of the earlier process of loss of final consonants. Once the final consonants appear, they are part of the process of devoicing.

In terms of stages, data from both Smith and Velten suggest that there are at least three stages in the loss of this process. These are given in table 12 with the examples from Joan Velten. In the first stage, final devoicing occurs. In the second one, vowels before voiced consonants are lengthened, even though the voiced consonants are devoiced. Finally, the devoicing process is overcome in stage 3.

Table 12   Stages in the loss of devoicing of final consonants in the speech of Joan Velten, adapted from Velten (1943)

Stages	Voiceless C		Voiced C		
1 (1;10)	nut wet goose	nat wut dus	mud red nose	mat wut nus	A. Devoicing of final consonants
2 (1;11 early)	nut wet goose	nat wut dus	mud red nose	ma·t wu·t nu·s	A. Lengthening of vowels before voiced consonants B. Devoicing of final consonants
3 (1;11 late)	nut wet goose	nat wut dus	mud red nose	ma·d wu·d nu·z	Loss of process of devoicing final consonants

(*2*)   In regard to assimilation between consonants and vowels, there are four possibilities. These are:

Regressive assimilation

i. C V   ii. V C
  →   →

(The arrow points to the element that causes assimilation.)

Progressive assimilation

iii. C V   iv. V C
  ←   ←

Each of these four possibilities has been noted in children's speech, although examples of regressive assimilation are more abundant.

(i) This case is one in which the child's vowel determines the preceding consonant. Jakobson (1968) mentions a case of this in the first stages of acquisition. He notes that at the earliest stages, 'many children are plainly not able to produce a labial sound before a front vowel' (49). The data from a child learning French showed the following forms: 'papa', 'dede', 'teter', 'de'. The last was used for the imitation of *be*, the bleating of a sheep. Oller (1973) has noted the same process in an English-learning child with a language disorder. The child had the following forms: *baby* [dɨdɨ] and *dog* [ba], showing the occurrence of the labial before [a] and dental before the non-low [ɨ]. Oller redefines the determining factor as one of vowel height. The labial [b] could only occur before a low vowel. A similar case has been noted by Dressler (personal communication).

Another process of regressive vowel assimilation has been noted by Smith (1973). He noted that [n], [t], [d] would all become velars when preceding a [u] resulting from a syllabic [l].

pedal	[b̥ɛgu]	(2;2)
beetle	[b̥iːgu]	(2;2)
bottle	[b̥ɔgu]	(2;2)

He states 'This is one of the most widespread rules found in children acquiring English as their first language' (14). This is a surprising remark as it is not substantiated by any data. Research will need to establish if this is true.

In discussing the data analysed by Ferguson and Farwell (1975), it was observed that after one child's initial 50 words a process of voicing appeared. This process is one in which consonants tend to be voiced if followed by a vowel. While Hildegard did not show this until a later period, Joan Velten (see table 3) showed this process from the beginning. Some examples are: *pocket* [bat], *push* [bus], *pie* [ba·]. This continued for several months for Joan, as shown by the following examples: *toe* [du] (1;9), *cap* [dap] (1;10), *soup* [zup] (1;9).

Voicing was also a common process for Smith's son A. It dominated his speech until 2;7, when it disappeared in a surprisingly short time. Below are some examples (showing loss of voicing in A (Smith 1973)) which show the sudden loss of this process:

telephone	'd̥ɛwiːbuːn	(2;2)	*television*	'dɛiːwidən	(2;6)
	'dɛiːboːn	(2;3)		'd̥eliːwidən	(2;7 early)
	'd̥ɛiːbuːn	(2;5)		'tɛliːwidən	(2;7 late)
	'tʰɛliːbuːn	(2;9)		'tɛliːwizən	(3;6)
tell	d̥ɛl	(2;6)	*pig*	b̥ik	(2;3)
	d̥ɛl	(2;7 late)		b̥iġ	(2;4)
	tɛl	(2;8)		b̥igiː	(2;5)
				b̥ig	(2;7 early)
				b̥ig pig	(2;7 late)
				pig	(2;8)

The examples show that the change started early in the month at 2;7 and varied somewhat before becoming more or less lost at 2;8. Thus the process may last for several months before being lost. For Joan Velten, voicing of initial consonants began to disappear at 1;11 and was nearly gone by 2;0.

(*ii*) In this case, the vowel alters towards some feature of the following consonant. One example of this has already been given in table 12, where a vowel by Joan Velten was lengthened if the following consonant was voiced. Another common case is the nasalization of vowels, where the vowel becomes nasalized before a nasal consonant. Leopold (1947, 209) noted that Hildegard, his daughter, did this. Genie, a child with severe language delay resulting from isolation, had examples of this as reported by Curtiss *et al.* (1974): *friend* [frɛ̃]; *dream* [drĩ]; *green* [grĩ]. This is a common assimilation. A third example of assimilation of vowels to consonants was Hildegard Leopold's process of vowel raising. A mid vowel was raised if followed by a [k], a sound made with a raised tongue. Two examples are *neck* [nik] 1;10, and *cake* [kik] 1;9.

(*iii*) Examples of progressive assimilation are less common. This would result in vowels being affected by preceding consonants. Leopold gives an example of this in the form *Bild* [bü] 0;9 to 0;10. The lip rounding of the [b] is taken over by the following vowel.

(*iv*) Here, examples are also sparse at this time. Leopold noted the form [ok] for *soap* at 1;10. He suggests that this may be the result of progressive assimilation, in which the backness of the vowel carries on into the final consonant. There is still much research to be done in isolating the various contiguous assimilations of young children.

(*3*) In discussing assimilation at a distance, Leopold has said, 'Assimilations at a distance occupied a much more prominent place in Hildegard's language and, I am tempted to generalize, in child language in general' (1947, 209–10). As with contiguous assimilations, noncontiguous ones may be considered both progressively and regressively.

Regressive	*Progressive*
V	V
C → C	C ← C

The most common regressive assimilation of this type is the assimilation of alveolar consonants to following velars. It has been called back assimilation in Ingram 1974a, and Velar Harmony by Smith (1973). Below are some examples from both:

Jennika		*A*	
talk	[kuk]	*dark*	[ġaːk]
dog	[gɔk]	*snake*	[ŋeːk]
take	[kek]	*dog*	[ġɔg]

Smith also noted (20) some assimilation of this kind except with labials in place of velars.

knife	[maip]	*stop*	[b̥ɔp]
nipple	[mibu]	*table*	[b̥eːbu]

Both, especially the former, appear to be common processes in the early part of this period.

Concerning progressive assimilations, Smith noted two that fall into this category. The first appears to be part of labial assimilation as just discussed. Alveolars would assimilate to a preceding labialized consonant.

squat	[ɡɔp]	*twice*	[ḍaif]
squeeze	[ɡiːḅ]	*queen*	[ɡiːm]

The second involves nasalization, and occurs only occasionally; a continuant would become nasal if preceded by a nasal consonant. Here are some cases:

noisy	[nɔːniː]	*nice*	[nait]
penis	[ḅinin]	*mice*	[mait]
smell	[mɛn]	*smith*	[mit]

Smith gives the forms in the second column to show that the rule is not operating for all forms.

(4) As with consonants, vowels can be considered for both progressive and regressive assimilation.

Regressive	Progressive
C	C
V → V	V ← V

The best discussion of these in the literature is that of Leopold (1947). Below are examples from Hildegard in which a vowel assimilates or becomes similar to a following vowel:

Handschuh	[haju]	1;10 >	[hauju]	1;11
Taschentuch	[hatu]	1;10 >	[hautu]	1;11
Hildegard	[hɪta]	>	[hata]	1;11
New York	[nɔjɔk]	1;11		

The German words occur because Hildegard is learning both German and English. The change in the first three examples shows that the assimilation occurred after the word had been used with appropriate vowels.

Leopold also observed progressive vowel assimilation. Here the vowel that changes assimilates to an earlier vowel in the word:

Loscher	[loko]	1;11
apple	['aba]	1;5
	['apa]	1;8

From these examples, Leopold suggests the following: 'These instances stand as examples for a certain tendency to give unstressed vowels a quality identical with or similar to that of the preceding stressed vowels' (212). This could represent a general process of acquisition, although further documentation is necessary.

These, then are some of the possible assimilations that children may show. Here they are summarized with examples from the text.

Table 13   Summary of some assimilations in the speech of young children

Type	Regressive	Progressive
CC	C C → Weakening of stops Labial assimilation *clock* [fwak]	C C ←
CV	C V → Height assimilation *baby* [didi] *dog* [ba]	V C ← Vowel rounding *Bild* [bü]
	V C → Vowel nasalization *friend* [frḛ]	C V or V C ← ← *soap* [ok]
CVC	C V C → Back assimilation *dark* [gãk]	C V C ← Nasalization *smell* [mɛn]
VCV	V C V → Reg. vowel assimilation *New York* [nɔyɔk]	V C V ← Prog. vowel assimilation *apple* [ʔaba]

Substitution processes   Lastly, even within the scope of one sound being replaced by another without reference to neighbouring sounds, there are some general processes that affect entire classes of sounds. Below are presented the major sound classes of English. For each, there are common trends in the manner of substitution by young children.

Obstruents			Sonorants				
Stops	*Affricates*	*Fricatives*	*Nasals*	*Liquids*	*Glides*	*Syllabics*	*Vowels*
p, t, k,	č, ǰ	f θ s š	m, n, ŋ	l, r	w, y	ḷ, ṛ,	i, ɪ, ɛ, e
b, d, g		v ð z ž			(h)	m̩, n̩	æ, ɑ, ə, ʊ
							ʌ, o, u, ɔ
							diphthongs

Obstruents   In fricatives and affricates, there is a frequent process of *Stopping*, i.e. replacing the sound by a homorganic stop. Below are some examples from A's speech:

safe	[deif]	(2;6)	*chair*	[dɛ]	(2;2)
zebra	[diːbrə]	(2;9)	*church*	[dəːt]	(2;2)
this	[dit]	(2;7)	*juice*	[dut]	(2;2)
shoes	[tuːd]	(2;9)			

Notice that examples like *this, shoes, juice* and *church* show the process in both initial and final segments. Although stopping drops out gradually, the manner in which this occurs will vary in degrees from child to child.

It is possible, however, to observe some general similarities in the way in which children acquire fricatives and affricates. Ingram (1975a) studied the use of initial fricatives and affricates in the speech of both normal and deviant children. The results indicate five general stages in the acquisition of these sounds. In Stage 1, children generally either omit the sounds or do not use adult words containing them. Stage 2 represents the widespread use of stopping for most if not all fricatives. If fricatives appear, they frequently vary in production. Stopping begins to drop out in Stage 3. Although some fricatives are replaced by a stop, most show a continuant sound of some kind. Sometimes this substitution is a liquid or a glide sound, (e.g. [s → 1]), although replacement with another fricative is more common. By Stage 4 most of the fricatives are produced correctly. A few of the more difficult ones such as [θ], [ð], and perhaps [z] will still be mispronounced. Stage 5 marks the acquisition of all of them.

The following are examples of each stage:

Adult sounds	Stage 1	Stage 2	Stage 3	Stage 4
/f-/	none	w	f	f
/v-/	none	v, w	v, s	v
/θ-/	none	d	t, ts, s	θ, (t)
/ð-/	(d)	d	d	ð, d
/s-/	(s)	d	t, ts, s	s
/z-/	none	d	r	none
/š-/	(s)	d	t, ts, s	š
/č-/	none	d	ts	č
/ǰ-/	none	d	d, dz	ǰ, d, dz
child:	Jennika 1;4	A 2;2–2;5	A 2;11–3;0	Anthony 2;4–2;6

The process of acquisition for these sounds is gradual and occurs over several years.

In the above examples with [š], [č] and [ǰ], the replacements were alveolar [t] and [d]. This is the result of interaction with another process that affects palatal and velar obstruents, called *fronting*. This is an early tendency to replace palatals and velars with alveolars. There are at least two separate parts to observe: (*a*) [č], [š], [ǰ] replaced by alveolars, e.g. [ts], [s], [dz] either without stopping, or as [t], [d] with stopping, and (*b*) the replacement of [k], [g] by [t] and [d].

Examples of the fronting and stopping of fricatives and affricates appear above in A's examples. The following are some of A's forms that showed fronting without stopping:

	š			č			ǰ	
shoes	[suːz]	(3;2)	chair	[tˢɛə]	(3;0)	John	[dzɔn]	(3;3)
shop	[sɔp]	(3;1)	chalk	[tˢɔːk]	(2;11)	juice	[dzuːs]	(3;5)
ship	[sip]	(3;1)	cheese	[tˢiːz]	(3;5)	jump	[dzʌmp]	(3;5)

These are later than the ones above and show how children gradually lose these simplifying processes.

The replacement of [k] and [g] by [t] and [d] is very common in young children's speech. At first it may operate in all instances of these sounds, and later be restricted to only initial or final sounds. Below are examples from Jennika in which it operates initially and finally, and some from a child observed by Hills (1914) who did this only with initial segments:

Jennika 1;5		Ruth Hills 2;0	
book	[bʊt]	cake	[teik]
dog	[dɔdi]	coat	[tout]
kitty	[dɪti]	go	[dou]
get down	[didəm]	big	[bɪg]

Nasals   The second large division of English sounds is the sonants which are most naturally voiced. With the nasals, the process of fronting will operate on [ŋ] and replace it by [n] at some point in most children's speech. Also, the entire class may be affected by an early process of *denasalization*, in which the nasals are replaced by the homorganic stops. Joan Velten at 1;10 showed this process in some of her words.

broom	[bub]	train	[dud]	rain	[wud]
spoon	[bud]	swim	[fub]	home	[hub]
jam	[dab]	room	[wub]		

This process does not appear to be an especially strong one, and some children may not show it at all.

Liquids   The liquid sounds in English are [l] and [r]. Edwards (1973) has examined the development of these in several children. My impressions indicate that there appear to be three stages in the simplification of these sounds:

Stage 1:   Stopping, (l), (r) replaced by (d)

Stage 2:   Replacement with a glide, [l] → [y] or [w]
$$[r] → [w]$$

Stage 3:   Replacement with a liquid [r] → [l]
$$[l] → [r]$$

Edwards does not deal with examples of the first stage and it may be a very early one in development. A showed some early cases of the process of Stopping.

lady	[ḍeidiː]	(2;2)	rain	[ḍein]	(2;2)
light	[ḍɑit]	(2;2)	rat	[ḍæt-]	(2;3)
lunch	[ḍʌt]	(2;4)	round	[ḍɑun]	(2;2)

The second stage is more common, and the one that children in some cases show over a long period of time. The [l] may become either [w] or [y]; children differ from one another in this regard. Edwards observed three children whose substitution was [y]:

Daniel		Eleni		Hildegard		
Lizzie	[yízi]	leaf	[yi]	look	[hek]	(2;1)
lookie	[yúki]	lion	[ya̤in]	lie	[yaɪ]	(1;11)
		light	[ya̤i̤]	like	[yaɪ]	(2;1)

Edwards notes that Hildegard also used [h], a sound considered a glide by some linguists. For [r], the more common substitute appears to be [w]. Here are some examples from Jennika:

rug	[wak]	1;9	*light*	[wait]	1;8
rock	[wak]	1;9	*lunch*	[wanč]	1;7
rabbit	[wædæt]	1;9	*lap*	[yæp]	1;11
			leg	[yek]	2;2

Some forms for adult words with /l/ are presented to show that Jennika passed through two substages. Before 1;11, all [l]'s went to [w], whereas after this time they went to [y], the pattern shown above.

The third stage is one in which one liquid is used for the other. Smith's son A had many examples of [r] being replaced by [l].

ride	[laiḍ]	2;5
right	[lait]	2;5
round	[laun]	2;5
run	[lʌn]	2;5

A clear case has yet to appear of [l] → [r]. Jennika showed this in a few forms such as *like* [rayk], but these were not widespread.

Glides Since glides are very early in appearance for most children, processes that simplify them are not widespread. However, glides occasionally seem to undergo a process of *frication*. That is, they are substituted by an available fricative. Velten's daughter Joan is a clear case of this for [y], which became [z]: *yard* [zɑ·d] 2;0; *yellow* [zɑ·wa] 1;11. This also was seen in words beginning with [l].

leaf	[zuf]		*like*	[zat]
lady	[zudu]		*lap*	[zap]

These show the application of more than one process, as discussed by Stampe (1972). In the latter, l → y → z with two processes involved—gliding and frication. Philip, a child observed by his mother Norma Adams (1972), had the following forms for [w]:

wheel	[vio]	2;0	*watch*	[vač]	2;1	*want*	[vɔnt]	2;2
whistle	[viso]	2;0	*why*	[vai]	2;1	*water*	[vadi]	2;2

These altered with forms with [w]. If [h] is considered a glide, it too underwent frication in the speech of Daphne at 2;4, as reported by Bateman (1916)—*house* 'souse'; *horse* 'sorse'; *hair* 'sair'; *hat* 'sa'. Although cases can be found, they do not appear to be abundant in number.

Syllabic liquids and nasals With regard to syllabic consonants, there is a frequent process of vocalization, which results in a full vowel being substituted for the syllabic element. Both Joan Velten and Philip Adams provide ample examples of this.

Joan (1;11)		Philip					
flower	[fawa]	cracker	[kaku]	1;7	apple	[abu]	1;7
hammer	[hama]	hammer	[mænu]	1;9		[apo]	1;9
table	[dubu]	flower	[favo]	1;11	bottle	[babu]	1;7–1;9
noodle	[nudu]		[fawo]	1;11		[bado]	1;10–1;11
bottom	[bawa]	bottom	[bada]	1;9			
pudding	[budu]	button	[batə]	1;9			
		lemon	[lɛmə]	1;10			
		open	[apo]	1;11			
		vitamin	[bada]	1;9			
			[bado]	1;10			

In Joan's case, the vowel that is replaced is assimilated totally to the preceding vowel. These examples are of Leopold's suggested process where unstressed vowels are assimilated to preceding full vowels. For Philip, there are several interesting points. For instance, [l] and [r] become [u], and later [o]. The nasals have an [ə] or [a] vowel at first, and then show the same pattern as the other syllabics, with forms with [o] around 1;10. This suggests at least two stages:

Stage 1:   Vocalization with assimilation, e.g. hammer [hama]
Stage 2:   Vocalization, e.g. hammer [mænu].

The second may even be marked in some cases with a change in the vowel quality before the syllabics are acquired.

Vowels   With regard to vowels, Miller (1972) has done an excellent study on the kinds of simplifying processes that affect them. The most common one is *neutralization*, where vowels are all reduced to [ə] (or [a]). Joan Velten showed this for all the following vowels at 1;11:[æ, ay, ɔ, ʌ, ɛ] before liquids and nasals. Aaron, the pseudonym of a language-delayed child observed by the author, showed widespread use of neutralization, as can be seen in these examples:

bed	[tʌt]	fish	[pʌsʌ]
belt	[tap]	teeth	[tʌf]
boat	[tap]	basket	[sʌkʌ]

In his speech, lax vowels appeared to be especially prone to undergo the process.

Deletion   Lastly, while all the processes above result in some simpler substitution for the various classes of speech sounds, the simplest process available is *deletion*. This is one that is common at the onset of acquisition, and is the first process available to the child. It is not unusual to see children delete segments before they attempt them. The use of deletion varies from child to child. A, for example, deleted certain fricatives before attempting them, e.g. *sun* [ʌn], [dʌn] at 2;4. It appears that individual children will use this process for sounds that are particularly troublesome for them.

Multiple processes   The above processes are among the most typical that operate on children's speech. While they have been presented one by one, it is important to realize that several may operate at the same time in a single word.

The child who says *pig* as [bɪk] shows several processes at once:

pɪg
b   Prevocalic voicing
k   Devoicing of final consonant

Once this is taken into account, children's reduced forms are much better understood. This can even be used to understand a child's words which seem quite unlike the adult word. Joan Velten, for example, used the form [bap] for *lamb*. Velten could not explain this form. Stampe (1972) points out that it is explicable once the multiple processes at work are isolated. Its explanation would be:

[læm]   *Adult form*
b   Denasalization
p   Devoicing of final consonants
y   Gliding
z   Frication
d   Stopping
b   Labial assimilation
a   Neutralization
[ḅap]   *Child's form*

While an extreme example, this shows that more than one process may be at work.

This concludes a relatively lengthy description of the phonology of the simple morpheme. As can be seen, several important aspects need to be taken into account: the development of perceptual categorization, the development of a phonetic inventory and the use of very general phonological processes. The result in progress towards adult performance in each of these areas is speech that becomes recognizable to strangers.

2.34 Completion of the phonetic inventory (4;0 to 7;0)

Since our primary interest is in the progress to the point at which the child has a good ability to articulate words, the discussion on this and the next stages of development will be brief. By this time the child has acquired a reasonably effective phonological system. This does not mean, however, that acquisition is complete at this point. There are still several years of active development ahead of the child. Relatively little, however, has been determined about these gains.

For one thing, the characteristics discussed for the preceding stage continue. The child still develops skills in processing longer words and sentences. Recent work by C. Chomsky (1969), for example, has shown the child's inability at this age to understand effectively certain sentence patterns. There are probably similar perceptual differences with longer words that are acquired. Examples of this can be found in children's singing of songs during this period. Jennika at 5;6, for example, sang the Jingle Bells verse 'bells on bobtails ring' as 'bells on cocktails ring.' Cases like this are numerous.

The phonetic inventory becomes complete during this period. That is, by age 7 or 8 the child can produce all the English sounds, including the fricatives and affricates (cf. table 6). At the same time, however, the tests showing this are based on relatively easy words. The child still shows difficulty in producing longer ones. When this occurs, many of the processes presented above operate. In Ingram *et al.* 1975, we studied the pronunciation of some more difficult words by children in this age group. Below are some examples of the kinds of mispronunciations that occur:

Child		*thermometer*	Child		*vegetables*	Child		*zither*
BB	(5;6)	[θəmánəbɽ]	BB	(5;6)	[véstəboz]	BB	(5;6)	[zízʊ]
ZG	(5;6)	[θɽmánətɽ]	BM	(5;6)	[véjəbḷz]	BB	(5;6)	[ðíðʊ]
BM	(5;6)	[θɽmáməpɽ]	JA	(5;7)	[béjdɔbʊ]	ZG	(5;6)	[zɪfʊ]
GS	(5;8)	[θámpətʊ]	GS	(5;8)	[vénčtəbḷz]	BM	(5;6)	[zɪsɽ]
RT	(5;11)	[θijámetɽ]	DG	(5;8)	[véštəbḷz]	GS	(5;8)	[ðɪsa]

Many of the children still showed numerous mispronunciations at age 6;0. Notice that for *thermometer* all the children have the initial [θ], but the word is still mispronounced. Thus, the acquisition of the phonetic inventory reflects just one part of the skills needed for adult speech.

Lastly, the child makes the first gains at this time toward the development of the morphophonemic system. Berko (1958) in a classic study with 5- and 6-year-olds demonstrated that children are just starting to acquire such alternations. She looked at, among other things, the development of the three plural endings and rules:

(1) –s after p, t, k, f
(2) –əz after s, z, š, ž, č, j
(3) –z after b, d, g, v, ð, m, n, ŋ, r, l, vowels, glides.

These are morphophonemic rules in that one morpheme (or meaning element) plural has three different shapes, based on the phonological environment. She found that children had acquired the rules for [s] and [z], but not the one for [əz]. This appears to occur in the next stage. Also, she showed that these rules are not just articulatory ones. The same three alternations are used for present tense and possessive in English, and children did better on [–əz] in those morphemes than for plurals. The difference here is that the child is not just learning phonetic patterns, but ones that are related to specific grammatical forms. Rapid development in morphophonemics, however, awaits the next stage with the onset of the ability to perform reversible operations.

2.35 Morphophonemic development

About the age of 6 or 7 the child begins to develop the ability to perform what Piaget calls concrete operations. When presented with a task to solve, the child will no longer just use a perceptual criteria for the solution, but will go back and retrace steps in trying to come to a better grasp of the situation. In phonology and syntax, this is manifest in important new developments. In Ingram 1975b, it is argued that many of the transformational rules that embed one sentence into another are acquired during this stage. As for phonology, the important step is the acquisition of morphophonemic rules.

Morphophonemics refers to phonological changes that result when one morpheme is added to another. Take, for example, the two words *electric*, *electricity*. The latter is made from the former by the addition of the morpheme *-ity*. Addition of morphemes will often result in sound changes. In this case, the [k] of the stem *electric* is changed to an [s]. The example of English plurals has already been touched upon. When the English plural [–z] is added to a word such as *church*, this results in a phonological process which inserts a vowel between the stem and plural, making the form [čȓčəz]. English has a number of complicated morphophonemic rules, many of which are discussed at length in Chomsky and Halle 1968.

Much of the growth of vocabulary during the years between 7 and 12 involves words of complex morphological structure. In dealing with these, the morphophonemic patterns need to be acquired. Two recent studies have shown very clearly that morphophonemic rules are acquired during this time. These are Moskowitz's (1973b) study of the rule of vowel shift, and Atkinson-King's (1973) study of the acquisition of stress contrasts.

English shows several patterns of vowel alternation where the vowel of some stem morpheme changes when a suffix is added. Below are shown three of the more common ones.

ay ~ ı		ey ~ æ		iy ~ ɛ	
divine	*divinity*	*explain*	*explanatory*	*serene*	*serenity*
collide	*collision*	*profane*	*profanity*	*obscene*	*obscenity*
line	*linear*	*grateful*	*gratitude*	*receive*	*reception*

Moskowitz (1973b) undertook a study to determine the acquisition of vowel shifts such as these. Two of the questions she sought to answer were, first, whether children have knowledge of rules such as these, and secondly, at what age they are acquired. She developed an elaborate study with several parts to be given to twenty-five 9- to 12-year-olds, nine 7-year-olds, and four 5-year-olds. One part of the study tested the above shifts in nonsense forms. The child was given a nonsense word and asked to give it back with the addition of the suffix *ity*. Below are some of the items and what would be the correct reponses

ay ~ ı	iy ~ ɛ
mayš > mıšity	kliyǰ > klɛǰity
fayp > fıpity	kliyč > klɛčity

The children, if wrong, were corrected after each item and success was determined by ten successes without error. Two other conditions were given (to the 9 to 12 year olds) which showed different vowel alternations. If children knew the rule for vowel shift, it was hypothesized that they would do better on the first condition than on the other two.

The results indicated that the 5-year-olds did not have knowledge of the vowel shift rule. With regard to older children 'there is no doubt that these children have knowledge of vowel shift, since the data are almost overwhelming. The differences among the results for the three age groups indicates that the acquisition of this information takes place gradually. Seven-year-olds and some 9- to 12-year-olds seem to tolerate any kind of alternation of vowel quality, while other 9- to 12-year olds tolerate only the major alternation pattern of English' (248). Moskowitz attributes the source of this knowledge to the learning of spelling during this age period.

A recent study by Atkinson-King (1973) also reveals major morphophonemic developments in this period of 7 to 12. She specifically studied children's knowledge of stress in regard to grammatical structure. Stress in English will vary depending on whether or not two words form a compound or a phrase. Below are some of the items that were tested in this study:

Noun compounds	*Noun phrases*
gréenhouse	green hóuse
rédhead	red héad
híghchair	high cháir
bláckboard	black bóard

These contrasts were tested by picture identification. For instance, the item *hot dog* would be given and the child would have to point to either a picture of a frankfurter on a bun or a dog panting in the sun. Other tasks were done to test these as well as other contrasts. For example, stress is also used to separate certain nouns from verbs.

Noun	*Verb*
récord	recórd
présent	presént
cónduct	condúct

These were placed in sentence pairs, e.g. 'Let's recórd his voice', versus 'let's récord his voice' and the child had to select the one that sounded best. Across all the various tasks and contrasts tested there were approximately 300 subjects between 5;0 and 13;0.

The results were generally the same as those of Moskowitz. This period appears to be the time at which these alternations are required. Atkinson-King notes in her abstract: 'In general a child of five does not yet show ability with these stress contrasts but one of twelve does; and the closer to twelve a child is, the more likely he is to have acquired it' (v). The acquisition of phonology, then, is not complete by age 7 but continues with the acquisition of more complex morphophonemic patterns.

2.4 Levels of representation

So far, the discussion of acquisition has proceeded with reference to two levels of representation: the adult word and the child's pronunciation. In between, it has been noted that a set of phonological processes apply to simplify the child's form:

Adult word → Phonological processes → Child's word

This assumption has also been made with regard to inventories of sounds that the child has or knows about. At the level of the adult word, there is an inventory of all the sounds produced in English. Meanwhile, at the level of the child's word, there is the set of sounds that the child actually produces. It is the latter that has been referred to in earlier sections with reference to the acquisition of a phonetic inventory.

It is possible to assume that this is all that needs to be taken into account in describing a child's system. Smith (1973), for example, takes this position in the analysis of A's speech. Since it is assumed that the child attempts any or all adult words, little attention is given to adult representation of words. The level of the analysis deals with the phonological processes of the child and the phonetic inventory. In fact, even the latter is more or less ignored so that the analysis comes down to an intricate discussion of phonological processes. Since the goal of these processes in this approach is simply to reflect the adult word, Smith calls them 'realization rules'.

This approach, however, ignores a number of basic facts about the acquisition of phonology in particular, and cognitive development in general. Perhaps the most striking one is that it assumes the child to be a passive creature in many respects, simply filtering the adult word. Piaget, however, has shown in his numerous studies that the child is far from passive, but is constantly acting upon the environment, and restructuring it in many ways. This view of the human being has led to a new term, structuralism, which describes this attitude toward the human mind. Piaget describes development in terms of the functions of *adaptation* and *organization*. The child needs to adapt to the world in order to develop and survive (cf. Flavell 1963, 44–52 for a useful discussion of these terms). To do this, the child actively organizes the knowledge it acquires.

Once these basic aspects of development are considered, the simplistic approach mentioned above needs to be revised. Piaget states that as the child develops, he is constantly achieving a balance between what he knows and what is new in the environment. This interaction between the child's mind and reality has two dimensions. The child is actively involved in the *assimilation* of the world to the structure of the child's mind. Also, as the environment continues to operate on the child, it results in *accommodation*, i.e. the changing of the child's structure to conform to reality. Both of these dimensions are necessary to understand the acquisition of phonology.

Imagine the child in the following situation. He is faced with acquiring the adult sound system. To do this the most basic part of this structure is taken into the child's mind. As part of the human function of *organization*, the child establishes or imposes structure on this. Development then proceeds through constant assimilation and accommodation. As the child takes a word and assimilates it, i.e. gives it structure, the child's ability increases and soon the child will need to accommodate, i.e. change the word to be more like the adult model. This can be schematized as:

Adult word → Child's system → Child's word

Notice first the need to consider the child's own system. The child acquires the adult system by creating its own structures and then changing these as the adult system becomes better known. The child's system is structured and will assimilate new adult words. For example, suppose the child establishes a basic CV pattern as a structure for new words. All new adult words will be assimilated to this pattern. At the same time, as the child learns more and more about adult words, the system will be restructured to accommodate to the adult words. Thus, it may establish a new CVC pattern.

The argument that the child has an active role in phonological acquisition is not a new one. Jakobson 1968 is the classic example of this approach. Jakobson argues that the child actively establishes contrasts between words. Others who have argued for considering the child to have its own system include Ferguson (1968) and Velten (1943). Those who oppose this include Stampe (1969) and Smith (1973).

If there is a need to consider a third level of representation in describing child phonology, the question arises as to what this encompasses and what it describes. It appears that the following need to be considered. The child is actively perceiving and producing speech. Both of these, then, need to be taken into account. Earlier, it was mentioned that evidence shows that children's perception is not complete, and consequently that it is not just a mirror of the adult word. The child's system of acquisition entails:

Adult word → Perception ← → Organization ← → Production → Child's word

Therefore, an accurate description of a child's phonology needs to provide information on *perception, organization,* and *production.* The rest of this section will briefly describe what each covers. The next chapter will use these and the processes discussed earlier to analyse a child's speech.

It is of course impossible to determine with any precision what a child's perception may be at any particular point of acquisition. As indicated in the discussion of the phonology of the simple morpheme, however, there are ways that perception can be reflected in a child's speech. For one thing, the child does not learn just any adult word. Rather, the adult words children attempt are usually simple in structure. The child's choice of words, then, reflects indirectly what a child perceives. Also, the child may have a preference for words with certain sounds in them. The observation of the adult words a child attempts will reflect to some extent the child's perceptual abilities.

The organizational level reflects the way in which the child is structuring the language. Since phonology deals with contrasts and attempts to assign one pronunciation to each morpheme, these are what the child strives for in learning the language. The description of a child's contrasts will be part of the organizational description of a child's speech. So too will be the processes by which the child arrives at them. Joan Velten, for example, at one stage voiced initial stops and devoiced final ones. The child's organizational system, then, did not have a contrast between voiced and voiceless stops. The process of voicing was operating between the child's perception and organization.

With regard to production, there will often be segments (or classes of segments) that the child alters purely because of inability to articulate. These products do not affect the child's ability to establish contrasts. They are part of the motor side of speech, and the fact that some sounds are difficult to pronounce. Pronunciations that are the result of production difficulties usually do not change in imitation, whereas organizational ones often do.

These, then, are three dimensions of the child's speech. An analysis looking at each will have the following parts:

Perception   — inventory of sounds and syllables in adult words
    $\updownarrow$ Processes
Organization   — inventory of sounds and syllables used contrastively
    $\updownarrow$ Processes
Production   — inventory of sounds and syllables produced

There are three inventories involved. The *first* would be of those sounds that constitute the sounds in the adult words the child attempts. While in reality this aspect may be omitted, it can be useful to see if certain adult sounds are preferred. Often initial vocabularies consist of adult words with primarily stops and nasals. This preference can often be determined by scanning the words. Also, it is worthwhile to examine the syllable structure of the adult words. If most are monosyllables, the perception may not be very advanced. The *second* inventory would be those sounds that are used contrastively. In younger children, this may be a small inventory. Those that are marginal would be so indicated in some way. The *third* one is the phonetic output, i.e. all the sounds the child actually produces.

Also, there are phonological processes to be specified. Although they can be given as one list, it is useful to divide them into categories that are purely phonetic or productive and those which are not. This will be exemplified in the analysis to follow.

There is a continuum between the simplest way to approach a child's speech and the more complex. The information above covers several aspects of a child's phonology, whereas the method sketched earlier does not. In several ways, the earlier method is the easier, but there is a real question of the extent to which the child's creativity is captured by this approach. There are times when one may wish simply to sketch a set of rules without considering the intervening level of a child's system. This should be done, however, with an awareness that it is only describing part of the child's actual system.

3

The analysis of a child's speech

3.1 The purpose of analysis

The survey just given of phonological acquisition in children provides the basis for the analysis of the speech of individual children. We can determine the general stage of development for a child, and then, within that stage look at the specific characteristics. Simply glancing through a set of forms of a child's speech can prove valuable in this regard. With experience, this kind of persual may be sufficient for determining the general nature of the child's speech. The degree of analysis will depend on one's time and purpose. The linguist is often concerned with a precise analysis, formulated within a formal system of rules. The clinician's needs are often not so precise, based more on the desire to determine the general inadequacies of the child's language.

While a survey of the sort just provided is the basis for analysing a child's speech, the actual analysis can be quite another matter. It is one thing to know something about some general patterns of speech and quite another to attempt to examine an actual speech sample with the purpose of preparing an analysis. The purpose of this chapter is to pursue such an analysis, going step by step from the first considerations to the final summary of the child's speech.

Since the purpose here is to provide a general impression of analysis to non-linguists, the analysis will be informal. Only a minimal number of linguistic formal devices is really necessary to analyse a child's speech effectively. At the same time, the analysis in some ways may be more precise and exact than individual clinicians and individual situations will require. While I characterize the child's data in several ways, only a few may be sufficient at times in actual clinical practice. Consequently, it is important to realize that the following analysis is *not an exact model* to be followed in every case in which one wishes to do phonological analysis. Rather, it is a *method* that is being demonstrated, a method which is adaptable to individual needs.

3.2 Ethel's phonological sample

In selecting a sample to analyse, I considered it appropriate to use data from a child with a language disorder. There are many analyses of normal children, but those of language disabled children are few in number. Since there is the serious issue of precisely how different the language of disordered children is from that of younger normal children, a normal sample might ultimately prove to be somewhat removed from the kind of language encountered in the clinical setting.

In examining several samples, it became clear that each differed in its own way. Each had some particular aspect that would be valuable for analysis and discussion. It was evident that none could be taken as representative of the 'typical' disordered child, whatever that might be. The one selected, therefore, can only be considered as a particular child's speech, which may be either very similar or very dissimilar to that of another child. The purpose of the sample is not to typify deviant speech, but simply to provide language for analysis. At the same time, it will provide a model for reference when issues of deviance and remediation are described in chapter 6.

Ethel is the child whose speech will be analysed. Her case is one of the few diary studies in print of a language-delayed child, reported by Hinckley (1915). Ethel was 5;6 when Hinckley first saw her in the autumn of 1911 when she entered kindergarten in New York City. Ethel gave the impression of a deaf mute, Hinckley claims, although it was eventually concluded that the child's hearing was normal. As for her behaviour in school, Hinckley states:

She showed an interest in what was going on by following it with her eyes and smiling pleasantly, but at the end of four months she had not said a word to teacher or child, nor had she voluntarily taken part in any activities. . . . (121)

Physically Ethel was oversized and walked with 'a lumbering movement, mostly of the hips—a spastic gait' (121). The ear cavity had a peculiar shape and the lower jaw protruded sufficiently so that the child could hold the tips of two fingers within the lower incisors. She had a three-year-old younger sister who was normal.

Hinckley soon determined that the child had no spoken language, and that she communicated primarily through various gestures and crude vocalizations. Hinckley began to work with Ethel after her adenoids and tonsils were removed in February 1912. She subsequently collected a sample of Ethel's speech as it developed over March, April and May of that year. This sample has been extracted from the article and is provided in table 14. Because Hinckley's transcription was inconsistent, it has been altered to a broad phonetic one. The table breaks down the speech into one-, two-, and three- or more syllable words. Within each, the items are also divided into the three months in which the data were collected. After each item is the day of the month that the item was recorded.

Several methodological observations are worth making on this sample. One problem is that Hinckley obviously was not a trained phonetician. Consequently the transcription is not very fine. It is possible, however, to determine the broad nature of each of the words, so that an analysis can be made. Since the transcription is suspect, this needs to be considered in trying to base crucial arguments on single examples. However, despite this, the sample has two very strong advantages. First, it provides the exact dates when all the forms were recorded. Virtually none of the recent analyses of deviant speech do this. In fact, most recent studies do not even provide the data on which the analysis is based. By not only providing data but also dates, it is possible to see *changes during a period of time*. As we will see, the child's speech improves in each month. Secondly, the data on Ethel shows her speech from the very first words to a vocabulary of nearly 200 items. It is the one

Table 14 Speech forms of Ethel collected in March, April and May of 1912. Day of month is in parentheses.*

One-syllable words

MARCH

beads	bi	(20)	come	tʌm	(27)	make	me	(27)	
big	ɪ	(20)	five	tay	(22)	red	wɛ	(20)	
blue	bu	(20)	four	tɔə	(22)	saw	dɔ	(27)	
board	bo	(22)	horse	ɔrt	(20)	stick	tɪ	(20) (22)	
box	ba	(20)	house	a	(27)	sweep	nθwi	(20)	
boy	bɔ	(20)	lines	lay	(27)	three	tö	(22)	
broom	bu	(20)	look	ʊ	(27)	two	tu	(22)	

APRIL

block(s)	ba	(25)	desk	dɛ	(25)	help	hɛ	(30)	
*blue	bu	(16)	door	dɔ	(25)	me	mi	(30)	
book	bʊ	(25)	dress	dɛ	(30)	*red	wɛ	(16)	
*boy	bɔ	(18)	girl	mʌ	(18)	shoes	tu	(18) (30)	
chair	mnæ	(16)	glass	dæ	(25)	sleep	ti	(30)	
	θæ	(25)	go	do	(30)	too	tu	(20)	
	θa	(30)	grass	dæ	(16)	up	ʌ	(30)	
cow	tæw	(23)	green	di	(16)	wake	we	(30)	
						yes	mɛ	(18)	

MAY

arm	ɔr	(21)	foot	tʊt	(9)	*make	me	(14)	stand	tæ	(9)
back	bæ	(7)	for	tɔ	(14)	*me	mi	(14)	string	tɪ	(14)
bank	bæm	(23)	*girl	dʌ	(7)	milk	mɪ	(14)	tail	te	(9)
bend	bɛ	(21)	gloves	dʌb	(7)	nail	ne	(7)	take	te	(2)
*big	bɪ	(23)	*go	do	(14)	neck	nɛ	(9)	tree	ti	(2)
*block	mba	(21)	goat	do	(14)	on	ɔn	(21)	*up	ʌ	(9) (14)
blow	do	(23)	good	dʊ	(21)	one	ʌ	(23)	walk	wa	(14)
	bo	(23)	*grass	dæ	(7)	pig	mɪ	(7)			
*book	mbʊ	(21)	*help	hɛ	(7)		pɪ	(14)			
bounce	bæw	(9)	hog	hɔ	(2)	plate	tet	(23)			
can	tæm	(14)	hole	o	(9)	play	te	(14)			
*chair	tæ	(7)	*horse	hɔrt	(2) (9) (14)	rake	me	(2)			
child	tay	(21)		hɔr	(7)		det	(14)			
*cow	mtæw	(2)	*house	æw	(2) (14)	run	wʌn	(14)			
dog	dɔ	(14)		a	(7)	sheep	tip	(2) (9)			
*door	do	(7)	jump	dʌmp	(9)	*shoes	tu	(9)			
down	da	(9)	like	day	(14)	*sleep	ti	(14)			
*dress	dɛ	(9)	*look	lʊ	(23)	stairs	tæ	(14)			

Two-syllable words

MARCH

Ethel	ætɛ	(27)	paper	pepʌ	(20)	ruler	muma	(22)	
Georgie	dɔrdi	(27)	pencil	pɛθ	(20)	table	te'ʌ	(20)	
Gracie	gwati	(27)		pɛmpʌ	(20)	wagon	wæθʌ	(20)	

APRIL

baby	bebi	(27)	pencil	pɛntɪ	(25)	Susie	tudi	(25) (30)	
button	bʌ	(23)		pɛntʌ	(30)	*table	te	(25)	
donkey	damθɛ	(23)	Polly	mami	(18)	*wagon	mæmʌ	(25)	
flower	pæwɾ	(16)		pa'i	(25)	window	mɪma	(25)	
*pencil	pɛmpa	(16)	stockings	ta'i	(30)	yellow	mɛma	(16)	
	pɛmp	(25)	Susie	mumɪ	(18)	Yetta	ɛ'a	(16)	

MAY

apron	ætn̩	(9) (21)	*Ethel	æta	(7)	put-on	puɔn	(21)	
	æpn̩	(9)	get-it	dɛtɪt	(14)		put	(23)	
blanket	dɔŋgɛ	(2) (9)	lion	layda	(9)	ribbon	ɪda	(9)	
	dɔmtɛt	(2) (9)	Lizzie	lɛtɪ	(23)	saucer	tɔtɾ	(23)	
		(14)	monkey	mʌmti	(9)	shovel	tʌ	(2)	
	bantɛl	(9)	nightgown	naydæw	(21)		tʌba	(14)	
	dɔmtɛ	(23)		namdi	(23)		tʌbda	(14)	
	bamtɛt	(14)		naynan	(23)	*Susie	tudi	(14)	
	bʌmptɛt	(23)	*pencil	pɛmpe	(9)	teapot	mima	(21)	
broken	bo	(2) (9)		pɛnθḷ	(9)		tipa	(21)	
	bɔptn̩	(14)		pɛntʌ	(9)	*wagon	mæmʌ	(7)	
carpet	tærtɛ	(14)		pɛntḷ	(14)	whistle	mwɪtɛ	(9)	
chicken	tɪtɛn	(2)	picture	pɪta	(7)		tɪpɪ	(14)	
	tɪ	(7)	pillow	pɪda	(7)		mɪtɪ	(14)	
	tɪ'ɛn	(14)		pɪta	(14)		ɪta	(23)	
*donkey	dɔmti	(14)	*Polly	pa	(14) (21)	wrapper	ætɾ	(21)	
dress-off	dɛtɔ	(21)							

Three- (or more) syllable words

MARCH

eraser	ʌbʌ	(22)	pick-it-up	pɪpæʌ	(22)

APRIL

butterfly	bʌ	(23)	handkerchief	æmkr	(30)
Elizabeth	mama	(16)	electric bulb	gæ	(25)

MAY

button-it	bʌtɪt	(23)	petticoat	k k tot	(21)
Christmas tree	tɪti	(2)		pɛpɪtot	(21)
	tɪtati	(7) (14)	piano	tæna	(14)
elephant	ɛmbɛ	(9)	put-it-up	pɪpiʌ	(9)
frying pan	tay pæn	(23)	Santa Claus	tæntʌ	(23)
*handkerchief	hæmtɪt	(21)	teddybear	tɛbɛ	(9)
			unbutton	ʌmbʌpa	(21)

* marks words that have already appeared in the sample.

rare diary we have of a deviant child from the first words onward. All modern analyses are samples of the child's speech in the midst of acquisition, with no record of how that point was reached. Data like Ethel's can be very valuable in comparing the early stages of normal and deviant phonological development.

Lastly, before the analysis is undertaken, it is important to mention that the data has been placed in tabular form in table 14 for purposes of exposition. It is not provided as the form in which data should be organized for a linguistic analysis. It is in this form here for purposes of presentation. In the next chapter, specific suggestions will be made on the organizing of data for analysis, as well as suggestions on other methodological problems of collection and transcription.

3.3 The analysis of Ethel's speech

The breakdown of the sample by the addition of *new* words at each month shows the following numbers:

	March	*April*	*May*	
Adult words of				
One syllable	21	20	31	
Two syllables	8	9	18	
Three syllables	2	4	10	
Total	31	33	59	123

Throughout, there is a predisposition to learn words of one syllable, although an increase in longer words occurs around May. The sample consists of at least one form from Ethel for 123 words, and two or more forms for each of several of the words. The latter is invaluable in observing how pronunciation of the same word will vary, even on the same day.

3.31 Ethel's stages

The first general question is to determine her overall stage of acquisition. Since Ethel is at the onset of speech, the first hypothesis would be that she would show characteristics of the phonology of the first 50 words. Since the sample shows twice as many words, two explanations are possible. One might be that she is in this stage, but is acquiring a much larger vocabulary because of the delay she has shown. The second is that Ethel has passed this stage more rapidly and that part of the sample represents the next step of development. A compounding issue is that in the normal child these two stages are separated by a different cognitive ability. Ethel, at age 6;0 would obviously be beyond the sensori-motor period and consequently would not be passing through two different cognitive stages in these three months.

In reality, all three of these aspects appear to be in operation. Since there is no cognitive parallel, the delay in vocabulary growth that occurs in normal children should not be a factor. Her acquisition of words shows this, since her vocabulary is developing fairly well. In the normal child, two-word utterances appear about the beginning of the fiftieth word. In Ethel's sample, two-word utterances begin to show about the end of April. At that point, she has 50–60 words. This compares well with the normal data. It suggests that the first period of phonology, that of the first 50 words, occurred in March and April, and that May marks the beginning of more rapid development. This is also supported by development in May, which shows an increase in two and three syllable words, and wider use of final consonants.

The overall picture appears to be as follows. Ethel shows in March and April many characteristics of the phonology of the first 50 words. She has a basic inventory of sounds and primarily CV words in her speech. In May there are indications that she is passing into the next stage, vocabulary increases, two-word utterances begin, and more complex phonological patterns appear in her speech. Also, since she is not progressing from one cognitive stage to another, there is no reason to expect a marked difference during the transition. In this light, the analysis that follows will examine the first two months separately from the third. These will be referred to as Ethel I (March and April) and Ethel II (May) respectively.

3.32   Ethel I

3.321   Syllables

As already noted, most of the adult words during this period are one-syllable, by a ratio of nearly 2 to 1. Perceptually, Ethel shows a preference for monosyllables. What about productively? Below are the basic syllable structures in her productive speech.

Ethel I syllables

CV	38	CVCCV	4
CVCV	11	CVC	2
V	4	Other	7

As can be seen, she has a definite preference for CV syllables. This agrees with the observations in the previous chapter that this is the dominant syllable of this period. An examination of the adult words reveals that there is widespread deletion of final consonants. Also, there is restricted use of the deletion of unstressed syllables which will be discussed shortly. Even the two-syllable words turn out to be restricted in structure. All the CVCCV forms are for one word, *pencil*. The CVCV have only two possible final vowels [i] or [a] (or [ʌ]). Thus, Ethel has a very restricted syllable structure at this stage, predominantly CV, and partially reduplicated CVCV.

3.322   Inventories

With regard to perception, each of the following segments occur initially in at least three of Ethel's adult words:

```
p   (5)      t   (4)
b   (11)     d   (4)              g   (6)
f   (3)      s   (6)              h   (3)
w   (4)                  y   (3)
```

These initial segments can be said to be salient ones for Ethel. To put it another way, an adult word that was monosyllabic and began with one of these segments is more likely to be attempted by Ethel than others. The segment [b] is most frequent, followed by [s] and [g]. This of course, is subject to that important condition, 'all other things being equal'. Compare this with the productive inventory for the four children discussed in 2.32, which is repeated below:

```
p   t
b   d
f   s   h
```

There is a remarkable similarity between these two, providing some evidence that the first sounds produced by young children follow an order similar to those first perceived, as suggested by Shvachkin.

Considering production, the consonants which follow were produced by Ethel in at least three forms. Forms are counted instead of words because the child occasionally pronounces the same word differently. The phonetic inventory of Ethel I appears below:

Initial		Medial	Final
p (8)	t (13)	m (6)	none
b (10)	d (9)		
m (10)			
w (3)			

Compared to normal data, the segments [p], [b], [t], [d] are predictable. The use of a fricative, [f], or [s] is missing and although [w] is mentioned as an early sound, the four normal children compared did not share it. [m] is used frequently, suggesting wider application by Ethel than the four normal children. Its use, however, is in line with Jakobson's claim that it is one of the earliest sounds. There is nothing particularly unusual about this inventory. Medially, only [m] is frequent, always occurring when preceded by another [m]. This suggests a phonological process of some kind, such as reduplication. There are no frequent final consonants and clusters generally do not occur.

Hinckley's transcription of vowels indicates that they are quite adult-like when in stressed syllables. Ethel does appear to have adequate ability with vowels and does not show the neutralizations to [i], [a], [u] shown by young normal children. This gives her speech a different appearance, from that of the young normal child. In unstressed (or second) syllables, however, there are restrictions. The only frequent vowels are [i] (or [ɪ]) (8 times) and [a] (or [ʌ]) (10 times). These suggest partial reduplication in the former and vowel neutralization in the latter.

Overall Ethel's consonants and syllables are like those expected in the phonology of the first 50 words, but the vowels are more advanced.

So far, I have presented two inventories for Ethel, the perceptual and the phonetic. The child's own organizational (or phonemic) inventory still must be considered. Basically we must ask this question—are all the segments shown in Ethel's phonetic inventory used to contrast meaning between words? This will be determined after an examination of the phonological processes found in the data.

3.323 Phonological processes

In observing the phonological processes in Ethel's speech, I will proceed by taking those discussed in 2.334 to determine whether they occur, and to what degree.

Deletion of final consonants This is a widespread process in Ethel I. Basically the process affects all final consonants in Ethel's words. It can be represented linguistically in the following way:

$$C \rightarrow \emptyset \quad / \_ \#$$

This states that C ($=$ consonant) goes to ($\rightarrow$), or is, deleted ($\emptyset$ i.e. zero) in the environment ($/ \_$) of the end of a word ($\#$). Another way to show this is that whenever $C\#$ occurs (i.e. a consonant at the end of a word), the consonant is deleted. Linguists use this format as a consistent means of showing how sounds change. It becomes particularly useful in showing sound changes which would be hard to conceptualize from a verbal description. Some examples of the process are:

broom	[bu]	*block*	[ba]
make	[me]	*desk*	[dɛ]
red	[wɛ]	*shoes*	[tu]

Deletion of unstressed syllables The deletion of unstressed syllables is infrequent, and the circumstances are not always clear. The few cases of deletion are:

pencil	[pɛθ]	*table*	[te]
button	[bʌ]	*rubber*	[ʌbʌ]

Otherwise, the unstressed syllable is reproduced in some reduced way.

Reduplication Total reduplication does not occur, but partial reduplication does occur in some forms where a final [i] is allowed.

Georgie	[dɔrdi]	*stocking*	[taʔi]
Gracie	[gwati]	*Susie*	[mumɪ]
baby	[bebi]		[tudi]
Polly	[mami]		
	[paʔi]		

This appears to be directly related to matters of perception. Words of two syllables will be attempted if they end in an [i] which allows for reduplication. In a linguistic analysis, the rule would be:

C, V, R* → 1 2 1 i
1 2 3

R* $=$ symbol indicating syllable that is produced by reduplication.

That is, words are reduplicated create a new syllable which contains the initial consonant and the vowel [i]. For example, *baby* would be considered as [be]R in the child's mind. Its production would be:

$$
\underset{1\ 2\ 3}{\underline{b\ e\ R^*}} \to \overset{b\ e\ b\ i}{\underline{1\ 2\ 1\ i}}
$$

The use of numbers here is simply a linguistic device to indicate how segments are repeated. Facility in using such devices, of course, is not a requirement for understanding processes like this; however, it can be a useful way of representing it. The occurrence of a glottal stop [ʔ] instead of the expected consonant results from the interaction of another process which optionally (i.e. not in all cases) deletes stops between vowels. It is returned to in the discussion of substitution processes below.

Devoicing of consonants Since there are virtually no final consonants, devoicing cannot be considered.

Reduction of clusters All clusters are reduced to a single consonant. These are always to the unmarked member, and indicate that she is in stage 2 of clusters acquisition (cf. 2.334). The only cluster that is permitted is nasal + obstruent sequences within words:

donkey	[domθɛ]	*pencil*	[pɛmp]
pencil	[pɛmpʌ]		[pɛntɪ]
	[pɛmpə]		[pɛntʌ]

Otherwise, the deletions occur in the predictable ways. [s] is deleted when followed by a consonant, i.e.

$$s \to \emptyset\ /\ \underline{\quad}\ C$$
stick [tɪ]
stocking [taʔi]

An exception to this, *sweep* [nθwi], may well be an advanced form (or progressive idiom), i.e. a form more correctly produced than others at the time. Liquids [l] and [r] are deleted when preceded by stops or fricatives:

$$\left\{\begin{matrix} l \\ r \end{matrix}\right\} \to \emptyset\ /\ C\ \underline{\quad}$$

blue	[bu]	*broom*	[bu]
glass	[dæ]	*three*	[tö]
block	[ba]	*green*	[di]

There are only a few instances of liquid + obstruent, but they are produced and suggest an early development that should be checked in the forms of the next stage.

horse [ɔrt]
Georgie [dɔrdi]

Assimilation   There are several instances where voiceless stops precede vowels. Except for the occurrence of *saw* [dɔ], these are never voiced.

pencil	[peθ]	*two*	[tu]
sleep	[ti]	*table*	[te]
stick	[tɪ]		

Prevocalic voicing is not a simplifying process of Ethel's speech. There do not appear to be any other contiguous assimilations. Also, noncontiguous assimilation is not striking, although this is limited by the restricted length of Ethel's words. There are, however, a few forms which suggest a process of nasal assimilation. These are:

wagon	[mæmʌ]
window	[mɛma]
yellow	[mɛma]

There is a substitution process in Ethel's speech (to be discussed) which optionally nasalizes glides [w], [y] to [m]. When this occurs, the medial consonant subsequently assimilates to [m]. This can be exemplified by the two forms for *wagon*:

wægn̩	*Adult form*		wægn̩	*Adult form*
wægʌ	Vowel neutralization		wægʌ	Vowel neutralization
wædʌ	Fronting		wædʌ	Fronting
wæθʌ	Lisping (optional)		mædʌ	Nasalization (optional)
			mæmʌ	Nasal assimilation

Both undergo vowel neutralization and fronting, common substitution patterns in Ethel's speech. After these two processes apply, [wædʌ] should occur. Ethel occasionally lisps stops and fricatives, and when this occurs [θ] appears. Lisping applies in the first form. In the second, however, occasional nasalization takes place and [m] is substituted. Once this applies, the nasalization persists throughout the word. Since the assimilated segment is always [d] (e.g. [g] → [d]; [l] → [d]), it can be shown as that in the rule which may be written as:

Nasal assimilation

d → m / #mV __ (where V = vowel)

The forms *Polly* [mami] and *Susie* [mumi] may also be a result of this, with the substitution process of nasalization extending to the stops [p], [t].

Substitution Processes   There are several general substitution processes, some which have already been referred to above.

Stopping   Fricatives and affricates are replaced by stops. This occurs in most cases and is also marked by additional changes in place of articulation.

five	[tay]	*saw*	[dɔ]	*shoes*	[tu]
four	[toə]	*Suzie*	[tudi]	*Georgie*	[dɔrdi]

These can be shown as:

Stopping
$$\left\{\begin{matrix} f \\ s \\ š \\ č \end{matrix}\right\} \rightarrow t \qquad \left\{\begin{matrix} j \\ z \end{matrix}\right\} \rightarrow d$$

The segments [t] and [d] replace all the fricatives. Given that they all become alveolar stops this suggests a very primitive stage in the acquisition of fricatives.

Lisping There are several occurrences of [θ] in the data. At first, one might think that the child occasionally can make adult [θ]. An examination of the words in which it appears, however, indicates that it is not the case. Rather it occurs for [s], [č], [d], [t] and only in a few instances for each. Notice that the normal substitution for [s] and [č] by stopping is [t]. This suggests that Ethel occasionally lisped the alveolar stops [t], [d]. The lisping rule would be optional; that is, it would only occur at times, not with every occurrence of [t], [d].

Lisping (optional)
$$\left\{\begin{matrix} t \\ d \end{matrix}\right\} \rightarrow \theta$$

The following are a few examples of this process interacting with others in words showing [θ]. *Wagon* has already been shown.

chair		pencil	
čɛr		pɛnsḷ	
tɛr	Stopping	pɛns	Syllable deletion
tɛ	Final C deletion	pɛnt	Stopping
θɛ	Lisping	pɛt	Cluster reduction
		pɛθ	Lisping

These do not represent steps in the pronunciation of the word. Rather, derivations like these separate the operation of different processes which in reality occur simultaneously.

Fronting This process occurs throughout the data. In all cases but one, *Gracie* [gwati], [k] and [g] are fronted to alveolars. This also affects palatal affricates which are stopped.

come	[tʌm]
glass	[dæ]
go	[do]
grass	[dæ]
Georgie	[dɔrdi]

(In several of the examples, the process of cluster reduction also occurs.)

Fronting
$$\begin{bmatrix} k \\ g \end{bmatrix} \rightarrow \begin{bmatrix} t \\ d \end{bmatrix}$$

The square brackets are used as a formal device to indicate that the change takes place straight across. That is, [k] goes to [t] not [d], and [g] goes to [d], not [t]. When braces are used, no claim is made about direction of change.

Glottal Replacement When a stop occurs between vowels, Ethel occasionally deletes the stop, using a glottal stop in its place. Hinckley does not use a symbol for it but her transcription suggests a separation between the vowels.

table	[teʔʌ]
Polly	[paʔi]
stockings	[taʔi]
Yetta	[ɛʔa]

The rule would be optional.

Glottal replacement
$C \rightarrow ʔ / V \_\_ V$ (optional)
Stop

This is the only general nonfinal process of deleting stops. There is only one case of the deletion of an initial stop, *big* [ɪ] so this is presumably idiosyncratic.

Liquid stopping and gliding Ethel differs in her treatment of the liquids [l] and [r]. The former appears to become predominantly a [d], although its phonetic form often differs because of either nasal assimilation or glottal replacement. It is also deleted in one form. Consequently it is difficult to say precisely what [l] is, except that it undergoes processes that stops do. Some pairs of these are given below.

	stocking		*Polly*	
Glottal replacement	stakiŋ		Pali	
	takiŋ	Cluster red.	padi	Stopping
	tatiŋ	Fronting	paʔi	Glottal rep.
	tati	Final c del.		
	taʔi	Glottal rep.		
Nasalization	*wagon*		*yellow*	
	wægn̩		yɛlo	
	wægʌ	Vowel neut.	yɛlʌ	Vowel neut.
	wædʌ	Fronting	yɛdʌ	Stopping
	mædʌ	Nasalization	wɛdʌ	Nasalization
	mæmʌ	Nasal assim.	mɛmʌ	Nasal assim.

Cases like this suggest liquid stopping:

Liquid stopping
$l \rightarrow d$

Examples like *line* [lay] and *look* [u] suggest it does not occur in CV structures.

The situation with [r] is a little more clear cut. Ethel substitutes [w] for [r], showing a process of gliding.

red	[we]	*rubber*	[ʌbʌ]
ruler	[muma]		

The only direct example is *red*. *Ruler*, however, provides indirect evidence. Recall that there is an optional process of nasalization which changes glides [w], [y] to [m]. If [r] becomes [w], it too should be a possible candidate for this process.

[rulr]	*ruler*
[rula]	Vowel neutralization
[wula]	Gliding
[wuda]	Liquid stopping
[muda]	Nasalization (optional)
[muma]	Nasal assimilation

The above derivation isolates the processes that would produce [muma] for *ruler*. The child's form for *eraser* also indicates that [r] may be deleted.

Gliding (preliminary)
r → w

Nasalization and deletion   The glide [w] appears in two words, *wagon* [wæθʌ] and *wake* [we]. In other words with [w] in the adult model, [w] undergoes nasalization, becoming an [m]. There are no phonetic instances of [y]. In the few cases where the adult word has [y], it is nasalized or deleted.

yes	[me]	*Yetta*	[ɛʔa]
yellow	[mɛma]		

There are two possibilities here. One is to have [y] as a possible segment, and assume it undergoes nasalization or deletion. Since it never occurs phonetically, however, this is probably an unjustifiable assumption. The second is to assume that [y] goes to [w], since [w] undeniably undergoes nasalization. Also, since [r] goes to [w] and may delete, it falls under that process also. This results in three general rules:

Gliding
$$\begin{Bmatrix} r \\ y \end{Bmatrix} \rightarrow w$$

Deletion (preliminary)
w → ø (optional)

Nasalization
w → m (optional)

The three can be said to be ordered in that each rule applies to forms having undergone the previous rule. *Yetta*, for example, would be explained as undergoing the first two processes. *Yellow*, meanwhile, would undergo the first and third. Forms from Ethel II support this treatment, as will be shown.

Lastly, [h] is deleted in the few adult words that have it, except *help*.

horse	[ɔrt]	*help*	[hɛ]
house	[a]		

The occurrence of optional deletion allows us to broaden the deletion rule to include [h], since they seem to be similar in this regard.

Deletion $\left\{\begin{matrix} w \\ h \end{matrix}\right\} \rightarrow \emptyset$ (optional)

Vocalization and vowel neutralization The last processes to be pointed out are those which affect the quality of final syllable elements. There are several cases of final syllabic liquids and nasals, and these undergo vocalization:

pencil	[pɛmpʌ]	*ruler*	[muma]	*wagon*	[wæθʌ]
table	[teʔʌ]	*paper*	[pepʌ]		

There are also cases of unstressed final vowels undergoing neutralization to [a], if they are not [i].

window	[mɪma]	(but)	*Susie*	[tudi]	
yellow	[mɛma]				

Since the phonetic reflexes of these two processes are the same, that of [a], or [ʌ], which appear to vary with each other, they can be combined as one process at this stage. Recall, however, that the data on normal children suggest that [u] and [o] are the common reflexes of vocalization. If so, we can state the two separately, assuming that the output of vocalization undergoes neutralization. Stating the change as two processes instead of one allows for predictions about later developments. Neutralization may drop out whereas vocalization may remain.

Vocalization $\left\{\begin{matrix} ḷ \\ ɾ̩ \\ ŋ̍ \end{matrix}\right\} \rightarrow ŏ$

Vowel neutralization
ŏ → ă
ă → ʌ (optional)

The latter can also have a second part, allowing an optional alternation between [a] and [ʌ] as suggested by Miller (1972). Since Hinckley's transcription of vowels is suspect, however, little can be made of this point.

3.324 The system of contrasts

Having specified the phonological processes, we can return to the question of contrast in Ethel's speech. The suggestion in 2.4 was to have three inventories: phonological, phonemic, and phonetic, with sets of processes between. So far we have the phonological and phonetic inventories, and one set of processes. The goal is now to determine those sounds that are used contrastively by the child, i.e. to cause a difference in meaning, and to separate those processes that lead to them from those that do not.

One indication that a process is not involved in contrast is when it is optional. There are several processes that come under this category. In unstressed syllables,

[a] varies freely with [ʌ]. The rule that optionally changes [a] → [ʌ] can be said to be noncontrastive in that the occurrence of one or the other does not distinguish one word from another. (The presumption is that words like *yellow* [mɛma] could also be found to be pronounced [mɛmʌ].) This is the case with lisping, glottal replacement, and glide deletion. In each case the rule results in free variation within a word rather than contrast between morphemes. Even if Ethel at some point should say *sleep* [θi] and *green* [di], the contrast in the child's system would still be [t] versus [d], in that the [θ] results from an optional process of lisping.

This is the case with nasalization, which optionally changes [w] to [m]. The alternation between the two forms for *wagon*, [wæθʌ], [mæmʌ] shows that it is noncontrastive. The resulting process of nasal assimilation is also noncontrastive as it is totally determined by the former. Even though *ruler* is phonetically [muma], for example, in the child's contrastive system it is [wuda]. As a result of this, it can be seen that the child's medial consonants are always predictable. There is usually [t] or [d], with the [m] the result of an optional set of changes.

Lastly, the nonstressed vowels in Ethel's speech are totally predictable, and therefore noncontrastive. In the forms where reduplication occurs, it is always [i]. In others, [a] occurs. Reduplication then does not result in contrasting segments. Both the consonant and vowel of the new syllable are predictable. Reduplication is therefore a noncontrasting process in this sense. What is contrastive is the fact that the word has a reduplicative morpheme. That is, the words *Susie* [tudi] and *too* [tu], differ in that one is CVR*, and the other is CV.

This results in a reduced set of consonantal contrasts in initial consonants only. These are:

p   t
b   d
m
w   h

Also, there are several possible contrasts in vowels, evidenced by forms such as:

stick	[tɪ]	*wake*	[we]	*go*	[do]	*blue*	[bu]
sleep	[ti]	*red*	[wɛ]	*door*	[dɔ]	*book*	[bʊ]

This results in the following use of contrasts in Ethel's speech:

(*1*)   Initial consonants contrast

(*2*)   Stressed vowels contrast

(*3*)   CV syllables versus CV partially reduplicated

(*4*)   CVR* versus CV $\left\{ {t \atop d} \right\}$ a.

The latter two show that the contrast is between two types of second syllables rather than the syllables within them. The rules and inventories for each of the three levels are summarized in table 15.

Table 15   A summary of the phonological anaysis of Ethel I

Perceptual level

Syllables—predominance of monosyllables;
2 to 1 preference over multisyllabic words

Segments—the perceptually salient initial consonants are:

$$* = \text{especially salient}$$

```
p    t
g*   d    g
f    s    h
w    y
```

Phonological processes

1 Deletion of final consonants: $C \rightarrow \emptyset \, / \, \_\_ \; \#$
2 Deletion of unstressed syllables (rare): syllable $\rightarrow \emptyset$
3 Reduction of clusters: $s \rightarrow \emptyset \, / \, \_\_ \; C$

$$\left\{\begin{matrix} l \\ r \end{matrix}\right\} \rightarrow \emptyset \, / \, C \_\_$$

4 Stopping: $\left\{\begin{matrix} f, \check{c} \\ s, \check{j} \\ \check{s}, \end{matrix}\right\} \rightarrow t$

5. Fronting: $\begin{bmatrix} k \\ g \end{bmatrix} \rightarrow \begin{bmatrix} t \\ d \end{bmatrix}$

6 Liquid stopping: $l \rightarrow d$ (optional word initially)
7 Gliding: $\left\{\begin{matrix} r \\ y \end{matrix}\right\} \rightarrow w$

8 Vocalization: $\left\{\begin{matrix} r \\ l \\ n \end{matrix}\right\} \rightarrow \check{o}$

9 Vowel neutralization: $\check{o} \rightarrow a$

Organizational level

Syllables: CV
              CVR*
              CV t/d a
              CV n/m t/d a

Segments:

```
C₁ = p    t        V = i        u
     b    d            ı        ʊ
     m                 e        o
     w    h            ɛ        ɔ
                       æ   a         ay
                                     æw
```

Phonological processes:

10 Nasalization: $w \rightarrow m$ (optional)
11 Reduplication: C, V, R*   1   2   l[i]
                    1 2 3
12 Nasal assimilation: $d \rightarrow m \, / \; \#mV \_\_$
13 Lisping: $\left\{\begin{matrix} t \\ d \end{matrix}\right\} \rightarrow \theta$ (optional)
14 Glottal replacement: $C_{stop} \rightarrow ? \, / \, V \_\_ V$ (optional)
15 Glide deletion: $\left\{\begin{matrix} w \\ h \end{matrix}\right\} \rightarrow \emptyset$ (optional)
16 Vowel neutralization: $a \rightarrow \wedge$ (optional)

Production level

```
C₁ = p    t    ?          C₂ = t/d
     b    d                     m
     m
          θ
          w    h
         (l)
```

Before leaving Ethel I, there are a couple of points worth noting. One is that she appears to have a rudimentary set of contrasts. This differs from the discussion of the normal child in which it was noted that it is not clear that one can talk of contrasts in the first 50 words of a child's speech. Since Ethel is older and probably beyond the sensori-motor period, however, it may be that she is capable of contrasts during these first words, as suggested by the early use of correct vowels. Also, it might even be that normal children start to use contrasts in this period. Research is needed on this particular point.

Also, it can be reiterated that one could analyse the sample here without attempting to establish an organizational level of contrasts within the child's system. Later, however, from the point of view of remediation, it will be argued that this distinction is quite important in helping the child to develop in therapy. Noncontrastive processes can be attacked first, since they interfere with the child's contrastive use of language. Also, once the contrastive sounds are established, remediation can systematically attempt to add to these in a principled way. Further discussion of these points is to be found in chapter 6.

3.33   Ethel II

The description of the phonology of Ethel I can be taken as a prediction about the nature of her words at Ethel II. That is, most of the new words should show patterns similar to those of Ethel I. At the same time, developments should be taking place. The following is a comparison of the language of Ethel in May to show the ways in which her system is changing.

3.331   Perceptual level

In Ethel I, monosyllabic adult words outnumber multisyllabic words by a ratio of nearly 2 to 1. In Ethel II, however, the number of new words that are multisyllabic just about equal monosyllables (28 to 31). The ratio drop in Ethel II is 1 to 1. In relation to segments, five addition segments appear initially in at least three adult words to increase those marked as perceptually salient. Below, these are added to the previous ones with squares around the new segments.

p	t	$\boxed{\text{k}}$
b	d	g
f	s	h
w		y
$\boxed{\text{m}}$	$\boxed{\text{n}}$	
	$\boxed{\text{l}}$	$\boxed{\text{r}}$

3.332   One-syllable words

In making a comparison between one stage in a child's grammar and another, a first step is to separate the *old words* from *new* ones. Velten (1943) has shown that new sound changes will often be found only in new words. Also, a glance at old words can show if they have changed in any way, and if so, how. A difference in pronunciation of the same word across stages will be a good indication of change.

Of the adult words with one syllable in Ethel I, 19 of these are repeated in Ethel II. Of these, ten are given the exact same pronunciation:

door	[dɔ]	*grass*	[dæ]	*me*	[mi]	*up*	[ʌ]
dress	[dɛ]	*help*	[hɛ]	*shoe*	[tu]		
go	[do]	*make*	[me]	*sleep*	[ti]		

For the other nine, the question arises whether or not they are outside the rules of Ethel I. These nine are:

	I	II			I	II	
chair	[θæ]	[tæ]		*big*	[ɪ]	[bɪ]	
cow	[tæw]	[mtæw]		*house*	[a]	[a]	[æw]
block	[ba]	[mba]		*horse*	[ɔrt]	[hɔr]	[hɔrt]
book	[bʊ]	[mbu]		*look*	[ʊ]	[lʊ]	
girl	[mʌ]	[dʌ]					

The first one, *chair*, is predicted by the rules. Recall that stopping was generalized to [č] even though there was no actual case of it. It was hypothesized that the [θæ] for *chair* resulted from stopping and then lisping. The form in Ethel II substantiates this.

The next three words, *cow*, *block* and *book*, at first appear to suggest a new process, one of placing an [m] before a consonant, which could be called nasal onset. A glance at Ethel I shows that there are two forms like this: *chair* [mnæ], *sweep* [nθwi]. Is there, however, the possibility that this process is actually part of one of the processes already formulated? A closer look at the data provides an affirmative answer. The most likely candidate is nasalization, since it also involves the production of [m]. Nasalization, as stated, is a replacement process, in which [w] is replaced by an [m]. Nasal onset, however, is one of juxtaposition. If nasalization is extended to include the cases of nasal onset, forms like *wagon* [mæmʌ] in Ethel I, would have to have the following steps:

wægn̩	
wægʌ	Vocalization
wædʌ	Fronting
mwædʌ	Nasalization (Revised)
mædʌ	Glide deletion
mæmʌ	Nasal assimilation

The postulation of [mw] as the possible origin of nasalization requires the use of glide deletion. This rule is already in the phonology, so that its operation here seems reasonable. There is, however, even stronger evidence for this revised treatment of nasalization. The forms of *whistle* in Ethel II are as follows:

> *whistle* [mwɪtɛ] [tɪpɪ] [mɪtɪ]

The sequence [mw] actually occurs, together with an alternate pronunciation with [m]. These forms, then, do not show a new process, but new instances of a former one, nasalization, which can now be revised as:

Nasalization (revised)
→ m / # __ CV (opt.)

i.e. insert an [m], optionally, before any consonant at the beginning of a word

This shows that Ethel has a general tendency to nasalize at the beginning of her words. This revised process will also explain the next form on the list, *girl*, where the nasalization 'overpowered' the [d].

The next two words, *big* and *house*, were idiosyncratic forms in Ethel I since [b] usually was not deleted and stressed vowels were usually not neutralized to [a]. Ethel II demonstrates these being regularized. *horse* shows the optional rule deleting [h] in operation, as well as final consonant deletion. The last word, *look*, is the only one suggesting a change in the earlier rules. Even in Ethel I, however, [l] → [d] was optional, due to the word *lines* [lay]. A look at other forms in Ethel II shows that it still is:

like	[day]	*look*	[lʊ]
lion	[layda]	*Lizzie*	[lɛtɪ]

The wide use of [l], however, does suggest the process may soon be restricted to medial position.

The old one-syllable words show the processes of Ethel I. What about the new ones? There are 37 new words, of which 27 (or nearly 2 out of 3) reflect the old phonology at work. Some examples are:

back	[bæ]	*play*	[pe]
milk	[mɪ]	*stars*	[tæ]
neck	[nɛ]	*take*	[te]

Some of these provide further substantiation of the previous rules. *Chair* [tæ], and *for* [tɔ] show fronting at work; *hog* [hɔ] and *hole* [o] show that glide deletion affecting [h] is still optional; [ʌ] for *one* indicates that this is also true for [w]. Lastly, the two forms for *pig* [mɪ] [pɪ] show the revised form of nasalization. To account for these two, as well as some of the others (e.g. *girl* [mʌ]) we need a new rule:

Consonant deletion (opt.)
$C \rightarrow \emptyset \,/\, \#m \_\_$

This is a production process, following nasalization, that deletes a consonant after [m]. It is optional, as shown by cases like [mba] *block*.

There are ten words that do not fit the rules:

arm	[ɔr]	*jump*	[dʌmp]
bank	[bæm]	*on*	[ɔn]
can	[tæm]	*plate*	[tet]
foot	[tʊt]	*sheep*	[tit]
glove	[dʌb]	*string*	[tɪŋ]

These show the beginning of the appearance of final consonants. The words *come* [tʌm] and *horse* [hɔrt] were hints of this in the first sample. These show that final consonant deletion needs to be optional for nasals and stops.

Final consonant deletion (revised)
$C \rightarrow \emptyset \,/\, \_\_ \,\#$ optional for nasals, stops

Since it still usually appears, it could additionally be marked by a percentage figure showing this.

The beginning of final consonants also provides a situation in which the child could begin to show assimilations of various kinds. Although more forms would be needed to substantiate them, there are two assimilations in the data. The forms for *bank* and *can* show that [n] goes to [m] after the vowel [æ]. This is a case of progressive contiguous assimilation.

Labial assimilation of nasal
n → m / æ __

The other assimilation is noncontiguous and occurs in *plate* [tet] and *sheep* [tit]. These should be [pet] and [tip] according to the rules.

Alveolar assimilation of stops

$$p \rightarrow t / \begin{Bmatrix} \# \_ V\, t \\ t\, V \_ \# \end{Bmatrix}$$

Two parts are needed to show the assimilation goes in either direction. The two syllable words *pillow* [pɪda] and *picture* [pɪta] show that the process does not occur across syllables.

3.333 Two-syllable words

There are only five old words of two syllables repeated in Ethel II. *Suzie* is [tudi] showing a repeated pattern, while *Polly* is [pa] twice, with a deletion of the final syllable. This could well reflect the loss of reduplication. Since final consonants and second syllables are beginning to develop segmentally, a straightforward rule to produce a final syllable would no longer be needed.

Three other repeated words are:

	I	II
Ethel	[ætɛ]	[æta]
handkerchief	[æmkɽ]	[hæmtɪt]
donkey	[damθɛ]	[dɔmti]

The word for *Ethel* is the same, except that final [ɛ] is now [a]. Nothing was said about [ɛ] in the first analysis but this alternation (and others in Ethel II) suggest that the unstressed vowel alternation between [a] and [ʌ] also includes [ɛ].

whistle [mwɪtɛ]
pencil [pɛmpɛ]

If so, it suggests a revision of vocalization and neutralization:

Vocalization (revised) $\begin{Bmatrix} ɽ \\ ļ \\ ņ \end{Bmatrix} \rightarrow \breve{ɛ}$

Vowel neutralization
$\breve{V} \rightarrow a$ (optional for $\breve{ɛ}$)

This not only accounts for Ethel II but also some unexplained forms in Ethel I, including *donkey*.

Handkerchief in Ethel I was an advanced form, i.e. it showed a pronunciation way ahead of other words in the sample. In Ethel II, however, it has come into the system and is simplified in the predicted direction.

hæŋkɾĕif	Adult form
hæŋkrtɪt	Stopping
hæntɪt	Deletion of unstressed syllable
hæmtɪt	Labial assimilation of nasal

The last process is introduced above. The form for *donkey* is further evidence for lisping, and shows the use of final [i] as would be expected. The unexpected cluster [mt] is discussed below.

The last repeated word is *pencil*

I		II	
[pɛθ]	[pɛmp]	[pɛmpɛ]	[pɛntl̩]
[pɛmpʌ]	[pɛntɪ]	[pɛnθl̩]	
[pɛmpa]	[pɛntʌ]	[pɛntʌ]	

All these variations show that Ethel has still not incorporated the word into her system. She appears to use different processes at different times as evidence for this failure.

In turning to new multisyllabic words in Ethel II, there are two structures from Ethel I that need to be kept in mind. There are two favoured types of basic syllable structure (or canonical shape) for Ethel I:

$$C\,V\begin{Bmatrix}t\\d\end{Bmatrix}a \qquad\qquad C\,V\begin{Bmatrix}n\\m\end{Bmatrix}\begin{Bmatrix}t\\d\end{Bmatrix}a$$

New words can be examined to see if they improve upon this.

Regarding the first, it is clear that it is still the dominant CVCV shape, in that [t], [d] are the most favoured medial consonants.

Ethel	[æta]	*Lizzie*	[lɛtɪ]	*chicken*	[tɪtɛn]
ribbon	[ɪda]	*picture*	[pɪta]		
wrapper	[ætɾ]	*pillow*	[pɪda]		
			[pɪta]		
		saucer	[tɔtɾ]		
		whistle	[mɪtɪ]		

In Ethel I, it was decided that [t], [d] were not contrastive medially, i.e. the distinction does not cause differences in meaning. The alternation between [pɪta] [pɪda] for *pillow* suggests that this is still true here. Also note that this confusion appears in the substitutions. It is not simply that [d] substitutes for voiced segments and [t] for voiceless. In *Lizzie*, for example, a [d] would have been appropriate. The pervasiveness of this pattern is evident in the form [layda] for *lion* where it is imposed where it would not normally occur.

For the first time, Ethel II shows some other medial consonants besides [t], [d].

apron	[æpn̩]	*shovel*	[tʌba]	*whistle*	[tɪpɪ]
	[ætn̩]		[tʌbda]		[mɪtɪ]
teddybear	[tɛbɛ]				
unbutton	[ʌmbʌpʌ]				

One could suggest there is now a contrast between alveolar [t], [d] and labial [p], [b] stops medially. The variations that occur in *apron* and *whistle* suggest that this is unlikely. Rather, what is probably taking place is what Ferguson and Farwell (1975) refer to as lexical contrast. The contrast may only be true between a few individual lexical items. Otherwise there is a great deal of free variation. The same free variations between these two positions occur in medial clusters.

The use of the second kind of shape with medial nasal + stop sequences is also frequent.

blanket	[dɔŋgɛ]	**donkey*	[dɔmti]
	[dɔmtɛt]	*nightgown*	[namdi]
	[bantɛl]	*elephant*	[ɛmbɛ]
	[dɔmtɛ]	**handkerchief*	[hæmtɪt]
	[bamtɛt]	*Santa Claus*	[tæntʌ]
	[bʌmptɛt]	**pencil*	(forms above)

Blanket, like *pencil*, appears to be unstable, not yet absorbed into the system. A curious part of these clusters is that [mt] seems to dominate, even though the two differ in place. One possible explanation is that the rule of labial assimilation of nasal may be the cause. This rule is most obvious with the vowel [æ] (cf. *can, bank, handkerchief*). Two exceptions, however, are *Santa* [tæntʌ] *frying pan* [taypæn] and *piano* [tæntʌ]. The rule could be broadened to other front vowels [i] and [ɛ]. This would account for some of the forms in *pencil* but not all. It would also apply in *elephant* [ɛmbɛ]. For *blanket*, it could be suggested that the rule applies before the process of vowel neutralization.

blanket	[blæŋkɛt]	
	bæŋkɛt	Cluster reduction
	bæntɛt	Fronting
	bæmtɛt	Labial assimilation
	bamtɛt	Vowel neutralization

The variations from the rule could be explained by the fact that it does not always occur.

There is, however, another possibility which works equally well. It would be a rule that changes non-initial [n] to [m]. It could be stated as applying most of the time, but not always. It would work as well as the above, and it is not clear how to choose between them. Instead, I will simply put both down as alternative possibilities.

Labial assimilation of nasal or nasal labialization (revised)

$$\text{(optional)} \quad \left\{ \begin{matrix} n \\ \eta \end{matrix} \right\} \rightarrow m \, / \left\{ \begin{matrix} i \\ \varepsilon \\ \ae \end{matrix} \right\} \underline{\quad} \qquad \text{(optional)} \quad n \rightarrow m \, / \, V \underline{\quad}$$

There is a third set of forms in Ethel II that reflects the onset of final consonants and the force of the CV $\left\{ \begin{matrix} t \\ d \end{matrix} \right\}$ a shape. These are two-word phrases that are used almost as if they were single words.

get-it	[dɛtɪt]	*button-it*	[bʌtɪt]
put-on	[putɔ]	*put-it-up*	[pɪpiʌ]
	[puʔɔn]		

These show that CVC words like *get*, *put* etc. have final [t] in the child's perception, but they are restricted to appearing if a word with a vowel follows. Otherwise they are deleted by final consonant deletion.

In Ethel I the treatment of the deletion of unstressed syllables is unclear. Here, the facts allow the possibility of refining the process. First of all, there are still cases where words are reduced to monosyllables.

chicken	[tɪ]	[tɪtɛn]
Polly	[pa]	
shovel	[tʌ]	[tʌba]

This is rare overall, however, so that two-syllable words now are by and large attempted. In reference to three-syllable words, there is more clear-cut deletion, although still optional.

button-it	[bʌtɪt]	*unbutton*	[ʌmbʌ́pa]
Christmas tree	[tɪti]	*piano*	[tæno]
	[tɪtati]		
elephant	[ɛmbɛ]		
frying pan	[taypæn]		
petticoat	[k k tot]		
	[pɛpɪtot]		
teddybear	[tɛbɛ]		

Generally, it appears that unstressed syllables are deleted in words with three syllables.

Deletion of unstressed syllables (revised)
Syllable $\rightarrow \emptyset$ / in words with three syllables

There are cases in Ethel II where the phonetic shape of the child's word does not directly mirror the adult word:

elephant	[ɛmbɛ]	*broken*	[boptn̩]
nightgown	[namdi]	*shovel*	[tʌbda]
lion	[layda]		

The first two show that the medial cluster [m] + stop is used where the adult word does not have one. The adult words do, however, have final nasals. There appears to be a perceptual schema here, in the sense used by Waterson (1971). The child notices that there is a nasal in the word, and restructures it to fit the shape used by the child for several other words. The words for *broken* and *shovel* show that the pattern is generalized to stops. *Lion* indicates CV [t/da] is a schema of this kind as well. Also, it is important that these [m] + [t]/[d] combinations are not clusters in the strict sense, but juxtapositions of two consonants across a syllable boundary. This is probably the preliminary step to the use of two consonants together in a single syllable. The fact that the nasals end the first syllable suggests that they will eventually be the first final consonants. This possibility, which has been suggested by Renfrew (1966), seems to be true for Ethel, based on the CVC words she has.

Lastly, there is just one new substitution pattern in Ethel II, the use of [b] or [v]. This is the first case of a change in the stopping rule. It is paralleled by [j] replaced by [d] in *jump* [dʌmp].

Stopping
$$\left.\begin{array}{c} f \\ s \\ z \\ \check{s} \\ \check{c} \end{array}\right\} \to t \qquad \begin{array}{l} v \to b \\ \\ \check{j} \to d \end{array}$$

Table 16   Revisions of the phonology of Ethel, based on Ethel II

Perceptual level

Syllables: acquisition of monosyllables to multisyllables drops to ratio of 1 to 1.
Segments: k, m, n, l, r, added to salient initial segments.

Phonological processes:
1   Deletion of final consonants: now optional for nasals, stops
2   Deletion of unstressed syllables: predominantly in three syllable words; optionally
3   (same)
4   Stopping: add v → b   ǰ → d
5, 6, 7 (same)
8   Vocalization: $\left.\begin{array}{c} r \\ l \\ n \end{array}\right\} \to \varepsilon$

9   Vowel neutralization: $\check{V} \to \check{a}$ (optional for ε)

Organizational level

Syllables: add CVCV as developing shape.
  also
  $\begin{array}{ll} CV & \left\{\begin{array}{c} t \\ d \end{array}\right\} a \\ CV & n \quad t/d \ a \end{array}$ operate as perceptual schemas

  Segments: C_1 (same) C_2 beginning of contrast
        V (same)   (t/d) v. (b/p), but not well established

  Phonological processes:
  10   Nasalization: → m / #__CV   (optional)
  11   Reduplication: may no longer be productive
  12   Nasal assimilation: now optional
  13, 14, 15, 16 (same)
  new 17   Consonant deletion: $C \to \emptyset$ / #m__   (optional)
  new 18   Alveolar assimilation of stops: p → t/ # $\left\{\begin{array}{c} \_\_ Vt \\ tV \_\_ \end{array}\right\}$ #

  new 19   Labial assimilation of nasal (or) nasal labialization

    $\left\{\begin{array}{c} n \\ ŋ \end{array}\right\} \to m / \left\{\begin{array}{c} i \\ e \\ æ \end{array}\right\}$ __   (optional) $n \to m / v$__   (optional)

Production level
    $C_1 : 1$ C_2 = add p/b

Table 16 summarizes the changes made in the phonology of Ethel, based on the words in Ethel II.

3.4 Analysis as a method

In concluding, it is important to return briefly to the point made at the beginning regarding the purpose of the above analysis. As one reads through it, there are times when one may want to question a particular judgement and may feel that an alternative is in order. Also, there may be counter-examples that one feels are sufficiently strong to negate the treatment. The distinction needs to be made, however, between the analysis and the method. The goal of this analysis is to show the method of analysis.

If one finds oneself re-analysing the data in this way, this shows the kind of thinking the linguist uses whenever analysis takes place. There are no set routines or procedures in attempting to analyse a child's speech. Rather there is the general goal of discovering the *most general rules* used by the child, based on what seems to be a phonetically plausible sound change. At first, these may not be immediately clear. For example, in Ethel I we have a rule changing [w] to [m]. This seems mysterious at first glance. Later, however, we see that the process is really one of using a nasal onset with words, and that this occasionally overruns the initial segment, especially if it is a glide [w].

The analysis demonstrates that any linguistic analysis is an active process, just as the child's system is an active one. It is difficult to say at any point that there is a right analysis. At every step, new insights may be gained through re-evaluating the same data or collecting new forms from the child. There is nothing inherently wrong with this. With each step we get closer to understanding the child's system.

Because of this, the analysis does not necessarily constitute a complete step before therapy begins. Rather, it continues with therapy and intermingles with it. The analysis is, after all, a hypothesis about the child's language. Based on it, therapy will systematically attempt to undo each of the simplifying processes. As therapy proceeds, new insights will be gained into the child's language based on what the child does and does not learn. At each step the method plays a crucial role, the method of comparing each word with the others to establish patterns of regularity.

Although general information about acquisition is necessary, the specific analysis of individual children also needs to be achieved. Each child will vary from others in its own way. This is particularly true with children who have a phonological disability. These individual variations can only be ascertained through the analysis of the child's speech into its dominant patterns. Such an analysis determines the perceptual, organizational, and production inventories of the child's speech, specifying the segments that the child hears, contrasts and produces, respectively. Also, there are simplifying phonological processes that need to be ascertained.

Any child's speech could be analysed in this way. Ethel is a child of approximately 6;0 with a reduced phonological system. She was not selected to represent any particular type of disorder, but as simply a child with a delay. Each child will show its own pattern. Also, the analysis is not meant to be the strict model for analysis, or necessarily the correct one. Each person will have different needs to satisfy in pursuing analysis. Some will wish to determine only the most general patterns, while others will want to do a precise analysis. The analysis presented falls somewhere in between. The emphasis of the analysis done is not only on correctness but also on the method of analysis. There are always alternatives one can suggest and pursue. What is important is that an analysis is a hypothesis about what constitutes a real pattern in the child's speech. It is thus an active pursuit which allows the change of rules upon the introduction of new data.

4

The methodology of data collection

4.1 Some methodological issues

In the previous two chapters there has been no serious discussion of the kind of data which was used. In chapter 2 a survey of acquisition was given without a treatment of the sources of data. Chapter 3 provided data from one child, Ethel, without much discussion as to whether the data really represented the child's language. There are serious questions that need to be raised about the kinds of information that can be used in examining a child's speech.

The major issue can be stated this way—what constitutes a representative sample of a child's phonology? First of all, the goal would be to have a text of everything the child has ever said, transcribed in fine phonetic detail, with an appendix of data regrouped in various ways to assist analysis. This, however, is an impossible goal. Instead, we have to be content with some sample or selection of the child's speech. There are several ways in which this sample could be faulty. It may not capture most of the words a child usually says. It may have been collected on a bad day when the child was not producing much. Also, it may not be transcribed properly, so that the symbols on the page do not represent what the child said. Or it may be just a list of words, when the child actually used each in a sentence with phonological changes caused by neighbouring sounds.

It is sometimes surprising that so little attention is paid to matters of this kind. Actually, if one wished, one could eliminate the entire data base of child phonology for deficiency in one or more of these aspects. To start, let us take the data from Ethel. There are approximately 200 forms given for a three-month period, many of only one occurrence. Are we to assume that this represents every word she spoke during this period? Probably not, for I think we can correctly assume that Ethel was using words throughout the period. What then, constituted the schedule of selection? In Hinckley's case it appeared to be everything said in her presence. Collections like these are never precisely given. Parent diaries, for example, never say more than that they are recorded whenever the parent is moved to do so. Outside observers often do not refer to any systematic schedule, such as an hour every week. We do not know what was said between samples and whether or not this information was significant.

Another aspect of this incompleteness is that of repetition. It can be shown that often children say the same word in a variety of ways. Many phonological diaries, however, only give one pronunciation per word. Velten (1943), for example, does this for his daughter Joan. Are we to assume that she was unique in this regard and never showed alternant pronunciations? It is more likely that he simply did not bother to give these, assuming they were mistakes of some kind rather than part of the child's system. What we usually get is what the observer thinks is a representation of the child's system. The aspect of repetition, in fact, has yet to be adequately faced in acquisition. Normal children will often repeat a word in long sequences, varying the pronunciation throughout. Little is known about these patterns.

This is also true of the use of words in sentences. In Ethel's sample the data is presented in the form of a list. In reality, many of the words were part of sentences. It may be that children show different pronunciation in sentences than in isolated use. In chapter 6 evidence is discussed that suggests this is true. The presentation of a list, which is usually done in phonological studies, completely misses this dimension of a child's language.

What about the use of an elicitation test, that is, a predetermined list of words as goals of elicitation? This is often used as a method of obtaining a representative sample of speech. This approach not only raises the above problems, but also misses a cross-section of words the child frequently uses. It may be that several of the listed words are unknown, or are known but not frequently used, or known but with an unusual pronunciation. This also introduces a number of problems about elicitation which are discussed in the next section.

Even if we are satisfied with what we consider is a representative sample, there is still the problem of transcription and recording. There is always an initial suspicion when a tape recorder is not used because the observer has to transcribe without the benefit of replay. Taperecordings were not made in most of the well-known diary studies. With or without recordings, there is also the question of the phonetic training of the observer. Hinckley, for example, was obviously not a trained phonetician. Even if the transcriber has phonetic training, there is the problem of whether he hears what he expects to hear. Recent evidence suggests that more than one transcriber may be needed for accurate transcriptions. All these aspects raise the possibility that the child's actual pronunciation may have differed from what was written down.

Besides hearing correctly, there is also the question of an appropriate phonetic alphabet. While there are phonetic alphabets available for use with adult languages, it is not always possible to use them to describe a child's speech. There may be particular modifications for which no symbol exists. There is a need for a phonetic alphabet with enough symbols to capture the various ways in which children articulate speech sounds.

No study of a child's phonology to date is totally free from criticism on one or more of these points. This does not mean, however, that none of the data is worth while. We usually assume the observer was accurate in his work, unless evidence appears that suggests otherwise. Nevertheless, it is important to be aware of the kinds of errors that can be made and how to avoid them. The rest of this chapter will discuss each of the relevant issues in the collection and transcription of data.

Even after data is collected and transcribed, there is still a third methodological problem. This concerns organizing the data both in preparation for analysis and for retention as a record of the child's speech. A final section will deal with some suggestions on how this should be done.

4.2 The elicitation of a phonological sample

4.21 The purposes of elicitation

Before we turn directly to methods of elicitation, it is necessary to discuss the reasons for the elicitation in the first place. There are two very general reasons for eliciting a phonological sample, for *screening* and for *analysis*.

The use of elicitation for screening arises from the desire to determine if the child's development is normal or not. In other words, screening is done to determine if a child has a speech problem. There are several stages involved in the process of screening a child. One step is to decide if the child is in fact slower than his peers. Once this is determined affirmatively, there is still the question of whether or not the child will spontaneously improve. It may be that the child will do so without special help. Screening, then, deals with the entire process of determining whether or not a child should enter therapy.

Analysis, on the other hand, is concerned with systematically examining the child's phonology for its own sake. The psycholinguist studying the language of a normal child does so to further his knowledge of the process of acquisition, not to determine whether the child is particularly slow or not. For the language clinician, the goal of analysis is specifically that of *diagnosis*. The clinician analyses the child's speech into its various patterns in order to diagnose the child's particular difficulty. While screenings reveal that the child needs assistance, analysis indicates specifically where the difficulties are.

There are many tests put forward to achieve these two goals of screening and analysis. Several of these are discussed and critically reviewed in Winitz 1969 (chapter 3). It is not the purpose here to examine all these tests and evaluate each. This would be of questionable value since most clinicians are more than familiar with many of them. What will be done, however, is a general evaluation of the goal from a linguistic point of view. Since the goals here are that of analysis, most attention will be devoted to this topic.

4.22 Screening

A first step in screening is the identification of the child with a problem. Investigations appear to differ with regard to the importance that is placed on this process. One position is that the only children who should receive therapy are those who are so obviously delayed that testing is hardly in order. This attitude is reflected in the first few sentences of a recent article by Compton (1970):

> In certain respects, the problems encountered in the diagnosis and treatment of articulation disorders may be paralleled with those encountered in the diagnosis and repair of a malfunctioning piece of electronic equipment, say a television set. For example, the TV repairman, like the speech pathologist, spends very little time trying to identify defective sets. Everyone can and does do this. (315)

This position is also reflected in the view that some children are given therapy because of a minor speech problem when they should not. The argument is that a child who receives such specialized treatment is identified as 'different' by his peers and undergoes an emotionally upsetting experience. This attitude is presented in a recent review article by Moskowitz (1972) of the book by Winitz (1969). First, Moskowitz is specifically concerned about children receiving therapy for errors in their speech which reflected dialect differences. 'I have met, for example, a child who was spending two hours a day of his summer vacation in speech therapy, rather than out in the sun: his "error" was the lack of differentiation of [ɪ] and [ɛ] before nasals' (491).

In a later passage in the review, she turns to the question of whether all children with speech defects deserve therapy.

> It is perhaps time for the goals of speech therapy to be seriously looked at and revised by the community of therapists. . . . Is it important or desirable that each child correct every possible speech error? . . . Many children can have slight defects trained out of them, with improvement for their chances of success in our society. But would our society as a whole benefit more by revising its attitudes towards 'misfits'? Indeed, there are many people with serious speech difficulties, and it is to these people that attention should be fully directed. (495)

Again, the emphasis is on restricting therapy to cases of severe dysfunction.

While such remarks by linguists raise important questions, they are unfair in at least two respects. First, there is the pragmatic issue of success in present-day society. As Moskowitz states, correction of minor speech defects leads to greater success in the sense of more jobs etc. If this is true, this can be a valuable aid to the individual involved. Secondly, a remark such as this implies that speech clinicians do not consider issues like these. In reality, there is a great deal of research on the question of what constitutes a population for therapy.

One line of research in this regard concerns the issue of whether or not children will improve spontaneously, without therapy. Both Roe and Milisen (1942) and Sax (1972), for example, have shown that children's speech will improve in time, even if it is delayed in some respects. There is the need to determine those children who will improve from those who will not. This is not easy.

This issue is often felt to be limited to marginal cases, that is, children who are in the stages of the completion of the phonetic inventory and that of morphophonemic development. There are also problems of this kind, however, with children in the most active period of development between 1;6 and 4;0. Both Compton and Moskowitz suggest working with children with obvious problems. There are, however, cases of children who are extremely late in starting language, and yet learn very rapidly without any need for assistance. A good example of this is reported by Nice (1925).

Nice had four children and followed the language development of each over several years. Table 17 gives the ages of the first word for each and the size of vocabulary at selected dates. While each child had a different rate of development, the third child, R, differed radically from the others. Although her first word was

Table 17 The date of the first word and the size of vocabulary at selected ages for each of Nice's children, taken from Nice (1925)

Child	Age at first word	1;6	2;0	3;0	4;0
'E'	1;2	145	—	1139	1765
'D'	1;8	—	—	856	1506
'R'	1;4	2	5	48	1135
'H'	1;3	9	155	804	—

at 1;4 she only had five words at 2;0 and only 48 by 3;0. At this point she showed a very delayed linguistic system. Suddenly at 3;2 she began to acquire language very rapidly until at 4;0 she had a vocabulary of over one thousand words.

Unquestionably R had a very reduced language system over the first three years. Despite this delay, Nice claims that she was a normal child with normal intelligence. Table 18 provides R's total language at three years of age. As can be seen, many of these are onomatopoeic sounds, e.g. *dog* [wawa] 2;0; *vehicle* [čuču] 2;2; *pigeon* [kuku] 2;4; *cow* [mumu] 2;8; *stop* [wo] 3;0. Nice says 'her language consisted of so many original expressions and derived meanings of obscure origin, that most of her associates understood little of what she said, and it was only due to careful study that I was able to ferret out as much as I did. . . .' (120).

Table 18 The speech of R during the first three years, taken from Nice 1925, with adapted transcription

1;4		2;4		2;8	
pig	[rr]	sheep	[ba]	rifle	[bu]
mama	[mama]	rooster	[kako]	deer	[da]
1;8		bear	[ur]	cow	[mumu]
bunny	[baba]	pigeon	[kuku]	where	[ha]
1;10		owl	[huhu]	good-bye	[ba]
hot	[ho]	banana	[nana]	2;9	
2;0			[ana]	not	[ʌn]
dog	[wawa]	I	[a]	on	[an]
2;1		don't	[da]	2;10	
horse	[ho]	well	[va]	grandma	[ma]
cold	[kr]	yes	[r]	2;11	
2;2		2;5		'hoo hoo'	[huhu]
(vehicle)	[čuču]	coal	[ko]	deer	[da]
toes	[rr]	I can't say	[rhr]	black	[ko]
doll	[baba]	2;6		3;0	
no	[na]	cocoa	[koko]	cry	[aa]
2;3		hurt	[hr]	like	[va]
(sisters)	[kugan]	other	[va]	stop	[wo]
fingers	[rr]	here	[hr]	3;1	
bicycle	[ho]		[krhr]	ant	[æʔ]
cat	[mnæw]	2;7		moon	[mu]
		bed	[čuču]	fall	[va]
		thing	[han]	have	[hr]
		near	[kr]	they	[hʌn]
					[hr]

Two further points are worth noting. One is that she was using this reduced vocabulary in sentences, so that she was beyond the holophrastic period.

[at	wawa	čuču]			'I (want to put the) dog (to) bed'
I	dog	bed			
[a	va	baba	čuču]		'I (see) another baby (in a) carriage'
I	another	baby	carriage		
[mama	an	čuču	baba	a–a]	'(if) mama (goes) in (the) auto, baby (will)
mama	in	auto	baby	cry	cry'

Her problem did not appear to be one of syntax, but of phonology. This phenomenon of a relatively developed syntax with a reduced phonology also characterized the speech of Joan Velten.

[za   nu·   but   wut   du·]
that   is   big   red   chair

The second point is that R's speech did not improve over this slow period.

... her pronunciation with one exception ('ba' which became 'boo-ba') had not improved one whit. ... In fact she wished us to use her expressions and her phrases rather than her learning ours. (120)

By age three, she presented the picture of a child who needed help. Later development, however, showed that she was capable of learning language on her own.

The above demonstrates that screening for language disorders is in many respects a difficult matter and one that raises many nonlinguistic questions. If one gives therapy to a child who may not need it, there may be psychological side-effects. At the same time, recent evidence shows that the earlier intervention begins, the better is the prognosis. A delay in beginning can also result in damage to some children.

Linguistics is not the discipline to provide the major answers to questions like these. There is another respect in which this is true. While linguistics is necessary to construct an adequate diagnostic test, it is not so crucial for a screening test. If the former is based on inaccurate assumptions, it will result in wrong judgement of the child's language. The screening test may be based on incorrect assumptions and yet provide results that do, in fact, predict success or failure. While a numerical score reveals nothing about a child's language system, it may reveal, through correlations with others, something about the child's comparative ability. The real contribution of linguistics resides in analysis.

4.23 Analysis

In elicitation of speech for linguistic analysis, there are three common approaches that can be used: (*1*) controlled elicitation through imitation; (*2*) controlled elicitation through naming; (*3*) uncontrolled elicitation through the collection of spontaneous speech. All three have been used in studies of acquisition, and most articulation tests make use of the first two.

4.231 The use of imitation

The most widely used articulation test (in America) is that of Templin–Darley (1960). This test elicits speech by giving the subject a predetermined list of words to imitate. In this chapter a number of serious questions will be raised about the usefulness of this test. The first concerns the use of imitation as a method of obtaining a speech sample.

The use of imitation assumes that the child will imitate words in the same manner that the child would produce them spontaneously. Templin feels justified in using imitation, based on the findings of a study she did in 1947. In that study she gave 100 normal children from 2;1 to 6;3 (mean age 4;1) articulation tests in order to study the difference between spontaneous and imitated productions. There were three tests: (*1*) Picture Test—the child was asked to name a picture; (*2*) Aural Test A—the child was asked to imitate a word with the picture of the object named before him; (*3*) Aural Test B—the child was asked to imitate the word without the aid of a picture. The same words were used in both aural tests. The results showed that there was no significant difference in any of the tasks. Scores were determined on the basis of the percentage of correct productions.

While these results indicate imitations do not differ from spontaneous forms, there are several reservations to be made. First, the subjects were all normal children. It may be that delayed children show a difference in this regard. Secondly, the scores only show correctness. A child could produce a particular word better in imitation than in spontaneous speech and still not be correct. For example, imitated [sɪp] *ship* would be better than [tɪp], even though they would be scored the same by Templin's criteria. These various points are not put forward to undermine Templin's study, but rather to understand the results in light of the several studies since that have shown that imitation results in better pronunciation.

Winitz (1969, 241–4) gives an excellent summary of several studies done on this topic. He cites studies by Snow and Milisen (1954), Carter and Buck (1958), and Smith and Ainsworth (1967), all of which have shown that children with articulatory disorders produce better when imitating. In summarizing his comparison, he states: 'In general the results indicate that stimulation results in an increase in the number of correct responses. . . . The increase is often small, however, and does not occur for all sound items. It may also be that effectiveness of oral versus imitative stimulation varies with such factors as age of the children, severity of the problem or differences in scoring method' (243). The result from group studies indicate that there is a slight difference between imitative and spontaneous speech at least with disordered children, and that the difference may vary from child to child.

Other studies with individual children further substantiate this finding. Faircloth and Faircloth (1970) tested this by specifically isolating on spectrographs nine words that had been both spontaneously produced and imitated by one child. The comparison between the lists shows that the imitated forms are closer to the adult model than the spontaneous ones.

Table 19   Spontaneous and imitated forms of nine words produced by a deviant child, studied by Faircloth and Faircloth 1970

	Adult word	Spontaneous production	Imitated production
1	*morning*	mʌ̀ː	mɔːnɪŋ
2	*bed*	bɛg	bᴱeɪd
3	*television*	tɛˀəʃən	tɛl'βɪgən
4	*daddy*	dɛdᵊ	dædɪ
5	*breakfast*	bwᴱ	bᵊwɛkʰə
6	*back*	bæː	bæk
7	*seven*	ʃɛvən	ɟɛvən
8	*Texaco*	teˡˀkou	tɛtʰɪkou
9	*sometimes*	kʌntaː	tˢʌntaɪⁿ

In unpublished research, I collected a sample from a 3;11 year old boy named Aaron who had a phonological disorder. The forms were produced by either naming a picture or imitating a word. The sample contained several words that were obtained under both conditions. These are listed in table 20. As with the child studied by Faircloth and Faircloth, there were several words that improved when imitated.

Table 20   Spontaneous and imitated forms of Aaron, a boy of 3;11 with a phonological disorder

Adult word	Spontaneous production	Imitated production
bed	tʌt	*bɛt
belt	tap	*tæwp
boat	tap	*pot
cup	pat	*kʌt
feet	pat	*fit
fish	pʌsʌ	*fɪs
letter	tato	*dado
meat	*mit	fwit
milk	næwk	*mæwk
paper	peto	*pep
spider	dʌdo	dʌdo
teeth	tʌf	*tif
water	dado	dado
basket	sʌkʌ (2x)	*bæskɪt
top	tat	*tap
dog	kak (2x)	kak
	gak	
	*dɔk	

* Indicates best pronunciation.

A last example of this difference is Genie, an adolescent girl who, because of being confined in a room for most of her life, had just recently started learning language. A report on her language by Curtiss et al. 1974 states the following about her imitative ability:

> Genie can pronounce many sound sequences in imitation which she does not use in spontaneous speech. It is clear that her output is more constrained by her own phonological 'realization rules' than by her inability to articulate the sounds and sound sequences of English. (534)

All these results suggest that imitation can lead to productions that do not reflect the child's abilities. They do not suggest, however, that imitation should never be used. Rather, they indicate that imitation may affect the output and that this should be kept in mind when using it, and that it should only be used when other methods are not effective. Later in chapter 6 we will return to the remedial question of whether or not words that improve on imitation are those that should be taught first in therapy.

4.232   The use of a single test item

A second problem with the Templin–Darley test concerns the use of one test word for each sound. The child is given only one word to produce in order to determine whether that sound has been acquired or not. Several points can be questioned here. Each relates to the fact that a child may produce a sound correctly in a word, and yet not do so on another occasion or in another word.

Templin bases her decision to use one word per sound on the study done in 1947. Besides studying the effect of imitation, she also wanted to see if pronunciation would differ from one word to another. To do this, she selected the following ten sounds to test in two different words.

Sound	Words		Sound	Words	
-ŋ	spring	ring	v-	valentine	vacuum cleaner
-t-	mitten	sitting	-z-	present	scissors
-t	feet	beat	-ǰ	cage	orange
k-	kite	comb	-i	feet	teeter-totter
d-	doghouse	doll	-ai	kite	bicycle

These were given as part of the three different tasks she used (as described above). There were then 3 × 10 or 30 situations in which the children could show alternation. The results showed only five of these in which there was a significant difference for scores for the pairs of words. From this she concludes, 'There is little difference in measured articulation when the same sound is tested in different words' (300).

There are, however, difficulties with this conclusion. They arise from her selection of test words, which is not very good for testing the hypothesis. First of all, since vowels are acquired very early by children, selection of them as test sounds is questionable. As for consonants, there are at least three reasons to suspect that pronunciation may differ from word to word. These are: (1) the syllable structure may vary, (2) the word itself may be unfamiliar, and (3) there may be phonetic elements in the word that create special difficulties. Templin did not take any of these into account when selecting her words. Except for the words for [d], all the paired words have basically the same syllable structure and stress pattern. All that her study shows is that children will not vary pronunciation between words when the structure of the words is very similar. It is still possible that other circumstances will cause variation.

In Ingram et al. 1975, we studied the ability of young children to produce word initial fricatives and affricates in words of varying structure. Among the structures were the following: (a) a monosyllabic word with a final fricative, and (b) a multisyllabic word with stress on the second syllable. These word pairs are presented in table 21. The children were asked to produce these words under three conditions: sentence completion, sentence recall, and imitation. Sentence completion would proceed as follows: 'This is a man; this is a fish. The man is catching the ____.'

Table 21 Percentage of correct productions on word-pairs of English fricatives and affricatives by children between 3;0 and 5;11 who produced both words

fish	(39/39)	100%	zees	(24/37)	65%
farina	(33/39)	85%	zucchini	(12/37)	35%
vase	(32/38)	84%	shelf	(33/41)	81%
volcano	(21/38)	55%	shampoo	(33/41)	81%
thief	(13/40)	33%	juice	(32/41)	78%
thermometer	(25/40)	63%	giraffe	(32/41)	78%
six	(28/37)	76%	chief	(32/35)	91%
safari	(24/37)	65%	chimpanzee	(25/35)	71%

In sentence recall, the child was asked to give back the entire sentence. While there were 73 children between 2;0 and 5;11 in the study, only the 41 children between 3;6 and 5;11 were given both members of the above pairs.

The results in terms of percentage of correct production show that there are a number of factors that need to be considered. The pairs for [š] and [j] showed no differences between words, a finding similar to Templin's. It suggests that for these words with similar structure the pronunciation will be the same. In each case the longer word was of two syllables long. In [s] and [f], there were slight differences, 9 per cent and 15 per cent respectively, in favour of the monosyllabic word. This trend increases for [č] 20 per cent, [v] 29 per cent, and [z] 30 per cent. These show that the pronunciation will be better in the shorter words. Lastly, the differences that occur for [θ] of 30 per cent show that other factors will interfere. The short word *thief* was much more difficult than the much longer *thermometer*. Most children tended to assimilate the [θ] to the following [f], saying [fif]. The results indicate that children will show different pronunciations of a sound in different words, depending on the phonological shapes of the words. Added syllables, stress, and assimilations can all affect pronunciation.

A second reason for rejecting the testing of the acquisition of a sound in just one word is that data from normal acquisition has shown that acquisition of sounds is gradual. Before a sound is completely acquired, it will fluctuate in correct usage, even within the same words. Because of this, testing a word just once will not reflect the child's real ability. A child may be at a point where he uses a sound 50 per cent of the time, but the testing of it in one item will show either 0 per cent or 100 per cent. In the above study, we had four sets of words and three tasks for each initial fricative and affricate, for ten pronunciations per sound. Many children showed variations as mentioned across the words and tasks. Below is an example of this from AC, a girl of 4;5 who varied between using [v] and the substitute [b].

Word	Sentence completion	Sentence recall	Imitation
vase	ves	bes	
village	vílɪj	vílɪj	ðílɪj
vegetables	véyəbļ	véyəbļ	béčəbʌlz
volcano	bəkéno	baykéno	

Notice that the use of [b] was not determined by the nature of the task. Each task had at least one use of [b]. This is also true of the different words. Each word except *village* showed a [b]. The factor that appears to determine use is variation; she is acquiring [v] but will substitute [b] about 50 per cent of the time.

Findings like these and the earlier ones on imitation cast grave suspicions on the use of tests such as the Templin–Darley for obtaining a representative picture of the child's phonology. Since this is the goal of elicitation in the first place, other alternatives need to be considered.

4.233 The use of naming

This method is a common one that is used to avoid the problems of using imitation. The Goldman–Fristoe Test of articulation, for example, is one that uses this method. Notice that this procedure has one main advantage over imitation, the elimination of the possibility of contaminating the results by providing a model. Its use has been widespread in constructing both standardized and nonstandardized tests.

There are, however, at least two problems with naming. One is a common one of getting together a set of pictures that will identify the word desired. This can often be a difficulty, particularly when the word is one that is not readily identifiable in pictures. The other problem is one that is not unique to picture naming, but also affects the use of imitation since both procedures test the use of words in isolation. As stated earlier, the use of words in sentences may influence their production. The use of isolated words creates an advantageous situation to the child and may not reflect his actual ability in conversational speech. Because of these difficulties, naming is by no means the answer to the elicitation of a child's speech.

4.234 The use of spontaneous language

The last common procedure is to collect a sample of the child's spontaneous speech. This procedure has been criticized for different reasons. Many children with a language disorder will be reluctant to offer any speech spontaneously. Also, a spontaneous sample does not provide a cross section of the sounds of English. It only gives those words the child happens to use in a particular context.

While the first criticism is real, and one which requires the use of elicitation, the second one is not necessarily valid. As stated in earlier chapters, the child selectively listens and chooses words that conform to the child's system. A spontaneous sample of sufficient size can tell a great deal about the child's preference for sounds. Those that do not occur may not just be due to chance, but to a selective avoidance on the part of the child. Also, a spontaneous sample provides words in sentences and often several words with the same sounds. Rather than one example of a sound, several forms are usually available. Because of these aspects, a spontaneous sample is not as unsatisfactory as some might think. Usually sounds that do not occur by chance may be so infrequent in the child's speech that their correctness is not important. Those that are important will appear in a number of words. A spontaneous sample can provide a general picture of a child's language that will be missing from samples obtained by most current tests.

4.24 Developing an analytic test

It is probably the case that, given the current state of articulation tests, the use of a spontaneous sample is the best means available today of obtaining a representative sample of the child's speech. This, however, requires ideal conditions. For one thing, most clinicians do not have the time to collect a very large sample of spontaneous speech. Also, there is usually little time to do a very detailed phonological analysis. Because of this, and the fact that some children simply will not talk, it is still necessary to develop a test that can provide an adequate sample of the child's speech. The rest of this section will discuss what is needed to construct such a test.

Winitz (1969), in a perceptive discussion of the inadequacies of current tests, suggests the following procedures (244):

(*1*) a constant set of stimulus words for all subjects;

(*2*) a particular sound should be elicited by several stimulus words;

(*3*) the method of elicitation (oral or pictorial) should be constant for all sounds;

(*4*) if possible, both methods of elicitation should be used (here he means spontaneous v. imitated);

(*5*) the criterion of correct production should be based on more than a single response.

Each of these procedures would need to be incorporated in our projected articulation test.

The first point refers to a constant set of stimulus items. Besides being given uniformly to all subjects, these items also need to be selected to reflect specific aspects of the child's system. Several years ago, acquisition was considered a process in which the child acquired individual sounds separately from each other. This is reflected in current articulation tests, which select a word to show each sound. As shown in chapters 2 and 3, however, acquisition is actually overcoming the various general processes that tend to simplify speech. These are processes like the deletion of final consonants, the reduction of clusters etc. Our test, then, will need to test specifically for the use of these. The number of processes given in chapter 2 would be a good list to start with. Testing fricatives, for example, would consist of a variety of items with fricatives to see how widespread stopping is. The choice of items would be geared to determining *which processes* are currently operating in the child's system.

In keeping with the second point, it would be necessary to test each sound in several words. In Ingram *et al.* 1975, we used four kinds of words: (*a*) monosyllables, e.g. *fish*; (*b*) two syllable words, e.g. *feather*; (*c*) three syllables with initial stress, e.g. *photograph*; and (*d*) three syllables with stress on second syllable, e.g. *farina*. These, of course, do not exhaust the possibilities. It is to be hoped that future research will help in decisions of this kind. Several words would allow us to ascertain how well the child has acquired each sound.

Third, the method of elicitation should be constant. This refers to the constraint of using one method consistently rather than several sequentially. This is to allow comparisons to be made. For example, if one child imitates a word, his production should be compared only to the imitations of other children.

The fourth point recommends the use of more than one method. In Ingram *et al.* 1975 we used a method that combined the strengths of both imitation and picture naming. This was the use of *sentence completion*. For example, a picture of a girl holding a vase would be used in this way: 'This is the girl; this is the vase.

The girl is holding the ——.' The child was required to supply the word. While providing a model as in imitation, the child still had to process a sentence between hearing the model and producing it. It was hoped that the intermediate processing would reduce some of the effect of straight imitation. Notice that by doing it in this fashion the problem of having the child identify the picture as in naming is avoided.

To check this, we also used two other techniques. One was a *sentence recall* method, where the child was asked to say the entire sentence. For example, after the sentence completion, the experimenter would say: 'Now, you tell me what's happening.' The last was the standard imitation task. With these techniques added, our projected test can draw on all or any number of these methods:

(*1*) Naming
(*2*) Imitation
(*3*) Sentence recall
(*4*) Sentence completion.

The fifth point proposes that the criterion of acquisition needs to be based on more than one response. In our study we had four words and three tasks structured in such a way that we had 10 items per sound, e.g.:

Type		Example	Completion	Recall	Imitation
I	monosyllable	*vase*	✕	✕	
II	2 syllables	*village*	✕	✕	✕
III	3 syllables	*vegetables*	✕	✕	✕
IV	3 syllables	*volcano*	✕	✕	

Each child's performance was then placed on a grid to reflect its design. For example, here is AC's production of [v] shown in this way (taken from above).

		/v/	
I	v	b	
II	v	v	ð
III	v	v	b
IV	b	b	
		50%	

Acquisition was set at 70 per cent. Even though AC had 50 per cent use, she had not acquired the sound. The grid does reflect that she alternated [b] with [v]. Scoring on grids of this sort will not only show the degree of acquisition but also the major substitutions.

If all these ideas are developed into a test, we would have a device that could elicit a representative sample of a child's speech. One immediate problem is that such a test would be enormous in size. However, this could be handled by the use of subtests. For example, if it was found that a child had trouble with fricatives, a more specfiic fricative test could be given, like that of Ingram *et al.* (1975).

There could, therefore, be a general test at first, then more specific ones devoted to delving into particular problems. The latter would only be used as needed. The construction of such a test would entail much work and effort, but it would be well worth the price.

4.3 Transcription

Once a method of elicitation is selected, there is next the problem of transferring the child's productions to a visual representation of it. If a child's speech is not accurately recorded, the analysis will fail regardless of how good the elicitation procedure is. There are two aspects of reproducing the child's words to a written system that need to be considered: (*1*) the area of recording and the process of transcribing, and (*2*) the phonetic system that is used in the transcriptions.

4.31 The use of audio taperecordings

The first question is whether or not the child's responses should be taperecorded. It is safe to say that this should be done whenever possible. The reasons for this are straightforward. By taperecording, the observer has a permanent record of the child's sample. This record can be referred to whenever needed over the weeks, months, or even years. The playing of taperecordings of a child undergoing therapy can demonstrate better than anything else how his speech has improved over a period. Also, the recording allows the observer to replay a child's utterances as many times as necessary to understand the phonetic characteristics. Errors that may have been made in transcribing immediately after production can be caught by replay.

Despite this, there are limitations in the use of taperecordings that need to be pointed out. The taperecorder needs to be of reasonable quality. If either the recorder or the microphone are not of good quality the tape will not be clear enough to catch the fine phonetic qualities of the child's speech. Even with good equipment, the conditions for recording need to be good. If the room is noisy or echoes, the tapes will pick up all of this, interfering with the child's speech. Even with good recordings it is still difficult to record accurately sounds which have high frequencies, specifically the fricatives and affricates. Since these are the most mispronounced sounds, it is important to be sure of the child's facility with them. Daniloff and Stephens (1974) have recently studied transcriptions of the production of adult /s/ by children. They compared transcriptions done from audio-tapes with those done during the actual testing. Even with optimal recording conditions, they found that the judges were more accurate in hearing the child's speech 'on site' than from the taperecordings. Results like this suggest that recording is a necessary but not necessarily sufficient procedure.

Another problem with the use of taperecordings is that it can lead to a certain amount of laziness at the time of actual elicitation. Since the child's speech is being recorded, the observer can become complacent about listening to the child's first-hand production. Inattentive listening would result from the attitude—'it's on the tape so I'll listen closely later'. The dependence on tapes has even led to the occasional use of one person to record the sample, and another one to transcribe it. Sometimes a long period of time may pass before the transcription is done. Both of these can cause errors. The observer should do an on-site transcription whenever possible, and use the tapes as a comparison. If tapes are used, they should be transcribed as soon as possible, otherwise the observer's memory will soon fade, and many of the utterances may not be identified in context.

While taperecorders should be used, this does not mean that a sample cannot be taken without one. One reason for this may be circumstantial. The observer may not own a recorder nor have one available. The other reason may be inherent in the nature of the child's language behaviour. A young child often may not speak frequently enough to allow the use of a recorder. In cases like this, the observer has to simply record the words whenever they are used. Otherwise the tapes will consist of huge gaps of silence. Even if the child does speak frequently, there is also the problem of the child's mobility. A young child will often move all over a room, reducing the effectiveness of a taperecorder. While this may be remedied by a wireless microphone, such equipment is expensive. Lastly, the conditions of the room itself may not be compatible. Templin (1957) in her classic study of articulation decided not to use a taperecorder because of the noisy conditions of the school where she collected the data.

In cases like these, the observer needs to do transcription on the scene. This has been done in most studies on phonology and has led to fruitful results. This approach has been criticized in that the observer may not hear a word correctly. Such a criticism, however, frequently reflects a misunderstanding of the context of children's language. Often young children will repeat a word over and over, so that any one utterance of it is not crucial. The goal is to establish the child's patterns, not to record every utterance made. In an elicitation list that requires ten productions of a word, the same result occurs. A sound may be misheard a couple of times, but the more cases there are, the less possibility there is for error. If necessary, then, it is possible to get a representative sample of the child's speech recorded without the use of a taperecorder.

4.32 The use of multiple transcribers

When speech is being transcribed by the observer, there is always the possibility that he or she may not be hearing the word objectively. This is always a problem since the process is entirely one of personal judgement. This may occur even if the observer has previous phonetics training. It is important, therefore, to be aware of this and examine the degree of error that may occur.

Henderson (1938) was one of the first to examine this question. In the study, which she emphasizes as preliminary in nature, three phonetically trained judges had to make independent transcriptions in three different circumstances. First, they recorded 'live' the responses of two third grade children with articulation problems. The children took a naming test containing items with all the English consonants. In the second stage, the same three recorded the speech of a five-year-old disordered child, the speech being amplified over a speaker to them in a separate room. Lastly, two of the judges transcribed an audio tape of the three judges' speech as distorted deliberately. Henderson then judged agreement between the judges on measure of correctness v. incorrectness and exact agreement.

There were two major findings of this study.

(a)   Correctness and incorrectness of consonants as articulated by subjects in person and in recorded speech possess a considerable degree of objectivity (1) when the judges have good hearing and (2) when the judges are practised and are expert in the detection of detailed speech sounds.

(b)   Fine distinctions of consonants, under many circumstances, possess a rather low degree of objectivity, but when the material to be judged is speech of a subject in person or speech electrically recorded, the articulatory productions are satisfactorily objective when judged by well-qualified persons. (356)

The findings show that a single observer can make objective judgements about correctness, but that there is variation when finer distinctions are involved. Henderson notes, however, that good training can overcome this.

A short study by Johnson and Bush (1971) looked at the issue of how transcribers may differ in recording finer phonetic detail. Nine participants in a phonetics workshop transcribed from an audio tape ten utterances of a child they had not seen. Below is an example of the variation that occurred with three pronunciations of *dada*.

Transcriber	dada 1	dada 2	dada 3
1	tʌdɔɪ	dadɔɪ	dædæ
3	tʰædæ^{l}	dædæ^{l}	dædʌ
4	t'adʌ^{l}	dæda^{l}	dædʌ
5	ʈʰædæ^{l}	ʈæʈɛ^{l}	ʈætʲæ
6	tadʌi	dada^{i}	dædæː
7	dæhdæʰɪ'	dæːdɛʰɪ	tɛʰtɛːʰ
8	ʈʰʌdaɪ	dadaɪ	dadjaɪ
9	t'ɛd'ɔɪ	dæðæ	

Transcriber 2 did not deal with these.

There are several things revealed by these transcripts. One is that variation will occur even between trained transcribers when fine phonetic detail is used, and when the transcriber is unfamiliar with the child. If one's interest is with understanding the child's basic pattern, one could attempt to eliminate some of the finer detail and make composite transcriptions: *dada* 1 [tæ/ʌdʌ^{l}] *dada* 2 [dæda^{l}] *dada* [d/tædæ]. These show the child has a [d] that varies with [t], and a low vowel somewhere between [æ] and [a]. Several instances of the word would eliminate much of the need to worry over individual transcriptions. A second point is that a consistent system of transcription needs to be developed. A standard transcription was also suggested by Henderson. Both studies indicate that the transcriber should be present with or familiar with the child and use a consistent transcription system.

Another factor that may affect a transcriber's judgement is whether or not he knows what word the child is attempting. Oller and Eilers (1975) recently tested this by having subjects transcribe the same words in two different conditions— one in which the subjects did not know the child's intended meaning and the other when they did. They found that knowing the intended word led to transcriptions differing from those when the word was unknown, and that the changes were phonetically more accurate. It appeared that knowing the intended word provided the subjects with a model against which they could compare the child's form.

All this research suggests that observers need phonetic training, and that more than one transcriber should be used whenever possible. Also, if there is a second transcriber, that person should be present at the time of elicitation in order to hear the utterances first-hand and become familiar with the child. If an observer has to work alone, it is important to keep in mind the problem of objectivity. This can be checked through relistening and not placing too much importance on any single utterance. The elicitation of several instances of the same word helps considerably in reducing errors in this regard.

4.33   The use of a transcription system

For many clinicians, the use of a broad transcription system (i.e. one not giving fine phonetic detail) will be sufficient. Such a system, however, is not precise enough to capture the finer phonetic details of children's speech. Even the International Phonetic Alphabet (1949) is not always effective because children utter sounds that cannot be captured within that system. To remedy this, Bush *et al.* (1973) have been developing a phonetic system specifically for children's speech. So far, they have devoted their efforts to specifying consonants. For those who are interested in finer transcriptions of children's speech, there is a summary of some of the main diacritics they have proposed in table 22.

The first part of table 22 presents diacritics of the IPA that have been found helpful in children's utterances. The second part gives diacritics specifically designed by Bush and others through a phonetics workshop. These are specifically developed for use in the description of consonants. First, some diacritics are given for the description of fricatives and affricates. A brief description of each is provided together with the sound for which the diacritic was especially developed. After these, there are some further diacritics developed for liquids and glides. Finally, diacritics are given for nasals and stops.

When first using a phonetic system, a broad system is usually more than enough. After a while, however, one begins to notice more details in children's speech. In many studies, these are called 'distortions'. One may begin to notice that the lips are more protruded than they should be, or that the sound is released with a pop. It is in an attempt to characterize more closely such distortions that diacritics like these have been developed. The diacritics in table 22 do not exhaust those provided by Bush and others. Rather, they are a selection of those that are more straightforward and can be understood without hearing. They are provided for the time when the reader finds that a braod transcription is no longer satisfactory, and wishes to develop the use of a finer phonetic transcription.

Table 22 A summary of some selected diacritic symbols for use in transcribing the speech of children, taken from Bush *et al.* 1973

IPA

Place markings e.g.			Voicing markers		
_	dentalized	s̲	o	Devoiced	b̥
<	advanced	<e			
>	retracted	e>	Timing markers		
^	raised	e^	:	Long	a:
v	lowered	ev	·	half-long	a·

Manner

ω	Labialized	f̫
~	Nasalized	ã
˒	Palatalized	t̡
ɩ	Retroflexed	t̢
ʰ	Aspirated	tʰ

Workshop markers for fricatives

ɵ	markedly spread lips, with orifice wide and shallow, [β̞]
↔	protruded, labialized and rounded sounds, [f]; [v]
m	heavily dentalized, [f], [v]
ᴅ	'wet' sound, an overlaid frication produced by saliva in area of articulation—all fricatives, e.g. [f] [s], etc.
⌒	Labiodentals released with noticeable pop, [f^] [v^]
⊥	Exaggerated protrusion of tongue for dentals, [θ] [ð]
L²	An alveolar sound produced more weakly, with lowered tip of tongue, [s] [z]
ʊ	marked grooved [s], [z], i.e. tongue is grooved more than usual, creating greater friction, [s̜] [z̜]
⊣	a palatal fricative with flatter tongue than usual, [ʃ̵] [ʒ̵]

Workshop markers for glides and liquids

ω̈	Exceptionally rounded lips
↔	Labially protruded [w]
ſ	A flapped [l]
l^	an [l] with a snap release, like that above for fricatives

Workshop markers for nasals and stops

⌒	snap release, e.g. m̂, n̂
↔	heavily protruded lips, [p]
L²	like above, marks a weakened t, with closure produced by blade rather than tip, [t]
ſ	a stop with fricated onset [fp] or release [pf] all stops with various fricatives, e.g. [tˢ]

4.4   Keeping a permanent record

After elicitation and transcription, the next problem to deal with is the system of organization of the data for both analysis and a permanent record. This is a problem which is not usually addressed in most articles, and yet it is a very basic part of any work dealing with data. If material is not organized in an easily manageable way, it will greatly affect the value of having the data in the first place.

4.41   Preparation for analysis

One purpose of organization is to prepare the material for analysis. While there are many ways that the corpus can be manipulated, there are two that are basic to all. These are a good copy of the original text, and an organized restructuring of the data for the purpose of analysis. Concerning the first of these, i.e. a copy of the actual texts, certain basic facts have to be recorded. If this is a spontaneous sample, it would need to contain:

(*1*) the child's utterance phonetically
(*2*) a word-by-word gloss of the utterance
(*3*) an interpretation of the utterance, if possible
(*4*) adult speech addressed to the child
(*5*) the context of the utterance.

For example, here is all this given for a young normal child who said *go there*.

Context	*Adult*	*Child*	*Gloss*
(child playing with puzzle)	What's that piece called?		
(child puts puzzle piece into place)		1 [gɔ da] *go there*	'it goes there'

Below the child's phonetic utterance is the word by word gloss in adult speech.

If the child is given an elicitation test, the same format can be used, although in a simpler way since the context is constant and the glosses are obvious. Usually the latter are simply the result of naming.

Context	*Adult*	*Child*
(application of test for fricatives)	These are people and that's a photograph. The people are holding the ____. What are they doing?	1 *photograph* 2 *holding the* [fótogræθ]

In this example, the child's speech is recorded in a simplified way. If the child's pronunciation is correct, it can be written in the adult spelling to show this. The mispronounced form in the second utterance will then stand out. In a case like the above, where a standard form is used, the record of the text can be made even simpler.

Item	*Sentence completion*	*Sentence recall*
photograph	(correct)	[fótogræθ]

The text will consist of the set of items and the child's production of each of the different tasks.

For an articulation test, the text may be sufficient as a record of the child's speech. With a spontaneous sample, however, a second step needs to be taken. This would be a copy of the child's speech with the *words given in alphabetical order*. This is done so that it is possible to look up any word or sound that is of interest. The data in table 14 of Ethel's speech is presented in this way.

There are important points to be kept in mind in putting the data in this form. One is that when forms are collected on different days, these should be noted. For Ethel, the date is shown. For example, *come* [tʌm] (27) means that the word was used on 27 March. Since Ethel's birthdate is not given, the data is shown by the date. More commonly, however, data is organized by chronological age. My daughter Jennika's diary, for example, is organized by month in this fashion.

Jennika	1;11	
*airplane	[ápeyn]	(24)
banana	[nǽna]	(14)
bandaid	[bǽndi]	(11)

Here is the beginning of the entry for the month of Jennika's life from 1;11 (1) to 1;11 (31). *Airplane* was recorded, for example, when she was 1;11 (24). The asterisk (*) indicates that it is a word that occurred in earlier months. The organization of the data into monthly periods allows one to collapse many forms and look at them at once, as in Ethel's analysis, for example. Ethel's speech sample shows that other considerations may lead one to group the data over a period of more than one month. Since a young child develops very rapidly, weekly groupings may be in order. By showing the data of each form, it is possible to keep track of changes that may be occurring over the month. Unfortunately, many people continue to give forms without dating them (e.g. Curtiss *et al.* 1974—data of Genie; Moskowitz 1970—data of Hildegard). Omissions like this make it impossible to observe changes over time.

Another point about the alphabetical listing by month is that it obscures the fact that many words are actually used in sentences. This was not shown in the table of Ethel's form. It can be done, however, in the following way. Ethel used the sentence [hɛ o dɔ] *help open door*, on 2 May. These could be entered in table 14 as:

help	[hɛ-]	(2)
open	[-o-]	(2)
door	[-dɔ]	(2)

The dash next to it would indicate the words which were part of a sentence and the side position of the dash would show the word order. Then, if there was something unusual about the forms, the context of the sentence could be examined in the original text to see if it may have influenced the words.

There are other ways that the data could be arranged. These include an alphabetical list according to the first sound in the child's word, or the same kind of list based on the final sound. The original text and alphabetical list, however, provide the two basic forms. With these two, the data is in a form for further analysis and manipulation.

4.42 Keeping a record

The organization of the data as mentioned is not needed just for the use of analysis.

It is also needed as a record of the child's speech so that progress over time may be observed. At the Institute for Childhood Aphasia, the following practice was used. Each child was sampled at the beginning of therapy. The sampling was done over several days to allow for the child's mood on any given day. The child was subsequently resampled at three-month intervals until he or she left the Institute. Each sample consisted of three different days.

	Sample 1	Sample 2 (3 months later) etc.
day 1	×	×
day 2	×	×
day 3	×	×

The same procedure was used at each sample period so that development over time could be observed. The practice of taking samples of the child's speech at regular intervals has also been encouraged by Compton 1975. Since the latter uses one elicitation test, naming, his sampling is done in one day. With a test of the kind described earlier, several days will be needed. (This assumes, of course, that the actual time testing each day is approximately between 15 minutes and 30 minutes.)

At the end of a child's period of therapy, a final summary of his speech over the sessions can be compiled. This would be a permanent part of the child's record. All the samples would be relisted into one alphabetical list showing the words across each sample. Here is an example of how this might look, taken from Jennika's diary:

Alphabetical list	1;10	1;11	2;0	2;1
...				
blanket	bʌdæt (10)	bʌkæt (8)	beŋket (13)	bɔkɛt (7)
	bʌdʌ (21)	bækɛt (14)		
...				

For each entry, the following columns would represent different sample periods and would show the pronunciations at each period (if one occurred). Although a final summary was not done for Ethel, the beginning of one would look like this:

	I	II (May)
apron		ætn (9) (21)
		æpn (9)
arm		ɔr (21)
baby	bebi (23)	
back		bæ (7)
bank		bæm (23)
etc.		

The record of a child who has undergone therapy for articulation would consist of all of the following: (*a*) audio tapes of each sampling, (*b*) the text of each sample, (*c*) an alphabetical list of the words in each sample, (*d*) the analysis of each sample, (*e*) a record of the remediation programme (to be discussed in chapter 6), and (*f*) the final summary consisting of a combined alphabetical list of all samples and how the words occurred in each.

5

The nature of deviant phonology

5.1 Defining 'deviance'

So far, several terms have been used interchangeably to refer to the phonological problems of these children—dysfunction, disorder, deviance, disability, delay. These have been used simply to refer to a child whose speech requires attention. In this chapter I will group all these under the term 'deviance' and try to specify what is meant by its use.

Assuming that our screening process has worked and labelled a child as requiring therapy, we can now ask several questions about the nature of his phonological abilities. First, we can ask if the sounds the child uses are part of a *system*. If a child's speech is largely unintelligible, we might tend to think the child does not put the sounds together in any systematic way. As section 5.2 will point out, the phonology of these children is systematic, even when their speech sounds largely like gibberish. The children are capable of rule-based behaviour, though it has not progressed to the same level as the normal child.

Secondly, we can ask if the child's system is in any way *different* from that of the normal child. To do this, we need to distinguish between a broad and a narrow use of the term deviance. The broad use of deviance is that of a general label for children who require therapy and who have no known organic basis for their difficulties. It is this broad use of deviance that has been used in earlier chapters, the title of this chapter, and in several recent articles (cf. Weber 1970, Morehead and Ingram 1973, Leonard 1973). In this sense it is a general label to refer to children who are not acquiring language in the normal fashion. The narrow sense, on the other hand, makes a specific claim about the nature of the child's system. There are two possibilities here. The child's system could be the same as the younger normal child's system. If so, we can say that the system is a *delayed* normal one. However, it may also be that these children acquire a phonological system in a unique way, showing patterns of acquisition that never appear in young normal children. If so, we can say the child has a *deviant* system. This in the narrow sense of the term, indicates that the child has a phonological system with different characteristics from the normal.

It is easy to see that knowledge on this latter point will be important in spotting children with disorders and planning therapy. If these children have unique characteristics in their language, these can be used to identify them. These characteristics also would be prime candidates for therapy. If, on the other hand, the system is only delayed, then the data from normal children will be especially useful in therapy. Forms can be taught in the order that the normal child acquires them.

In what follows, the broad sense of deviant will be used with reference to these children and their phonologies. Deviant children, therefore, are simply children who require therapy, and deviant phonology refers to the study of the phonology of these children. The narrow sense of deviance will be restricted to the phrase *deviant system*. This refers to the hypothesis that these children have unique phonological systems. The question 'do deviant children have deviant systems?' shows both uses of the term. Section 5.3 will attempt to answer this question.

Thirdly, questions about systematic phonology and deviant systems can be asked individually for specific disorders with an organic basis. Are there unique characteristics that distinguish hard-of-hearing, cleft palate, mongoloid, and mentally retarded children? Section 5.4 reviews the research to date on the phonologies of children suffering from each of these disorders. Much of the discussion before that section will be referring to children who have none of these disorders, but still show phonological dysfunction. They are traditionally referred to as having functional articulation disorders. While this covers a wide diversity of difficulties it is often even harder to try to narrow this group more than this.

5.2 The systematic nature of deviant phonology

Virtually every study that has undertaken the linguistic analysis of a child with a phonological disability has revealed system in the child's speech. This is true both for children with a general disorder and those with specific syndromes (e.g. hard-of-hearing, cleft palate etc.) Table 23 presents information about some deviant children whose phonology has been linguistically analysed.

Table 23   Sources of linguistic analyses of children with phonological disability

Child	Age	Character of data	Investigator(s)
Ethel	6;0–6;2	Diary of approx. 200 words over 3-month period	Hinckley 1915
Kevin	6;6	Spontaneous text of 43 words	Haas 1963
Tom	6;0	Elicitation of approx. 100 words through naming	Compton 1970
Jim	4;6		
Frank	5;0 to ?	above procedure, given initially at 5;0 and again 6 times (time of intervals not given)	Compton 1975
BN (boy)	5;2, 5;8, 6;3	Elicitation of unstated number of words through naming, and sample of spontaneous speech. Procedure followed at 3 ages	Pollock and Rees 1972
Val	Exact ages not given—between	Photo Articulation Test (PAT) (Pendergast et al. 1965).	Oller et al. 1972. Summarized in Oller 1973
Jean	given—between	Elicitation through imitation of test	
Vince	3;8 and 5;11	words in Fairbanks 1940	
Jay		PAT and imitation of words of Goldman–Fristoe Test of Articulation	
Curt		Unknown	
Bernie	3;3	Elicitation of unstated number of words through naming	Edwards and Bernhardt 1973a
Marc	3;3		
Jennifer	4;4		
Christina	5;3		
Joe	4;6	Elicitation procedure not given (spontaneous sample?); size unknown but several examples given	Lorentz 1972, 1974
David	4;0		

These studies in their individual ways demonstrate that deviant children have systematic ways of using sounds to produce words. Most do this by identifying the phonological processes that simplify the adult words. The studies are also similar in the way in which the data have been collected. Most use a naming procedure of some kind, either standardized or of their own design. This procedure is subject to the criticism already mentioned. Also, unfortunately, most give rules rather than examples of the child's words, so that few data are actually provided. This is particularly true of the studies by Compton and Oller. Because of this, it is difficult to get a feel for the way the children produced words. Fortunately the studies by Edwards and Bernhardt and by Lorentz provide several examples for the rules they give so that their analyses can be justified. An analysis can be accepted or rejected only on the basis of the actual data.

5.21   Kevin

Hinckley 1915 was one of the first reports on the language of a deviant child. This data has already been analysed in detail in chapter 3. A glance at that chapter will show the systematic processes and contrasts the child used in its language. Several years elapsed before another report on a deviant child appeared. In 1963 Haas provided a linguistic analysis of a six-and-a-half-year old boy Kevin. One striking characteristic of this analysis is that it is based on an amazingly small corpus. Even so, Haas was able to throw considerable light on the child's system. 'His mistakes, though many and varied, seem to be selective and systematic' (Haas, 240).

Kevin's language is more advanced than Ethel's in several ways. First, he uses much longer sentences, e.g. *once upon a time was little green fish with so many friends.* He had been able to develop grammatically despite his speech defect. Secondly, he uses many final consonants whereas Ethel had not begun to use them widely.

Kevin	[teɫʷin]	*was*	[wəz̥]	*up*	[ʔɒp]
once	[wʌns]	*green*	[tiːn]	*good*	[dud]
time	[taim]	*fish*	[ḍiθ]		

Even the word that shows loss, *big* [ḍi], also shows knowledge of the final consonant in *bigger* [biḍə]. Although a small sample it suggests that the child had a rather large vocabulary compared to Ethel.

At the same time, Kevin's speech, like Ethel's, shows the systematic use of phonological processes and contrasts. Kevin's phonetic and phonemic inventories of consonants are:

Phonetic inventory		*Phonemic inventory*	
p	t, d	p	t
m	n	m	n
	θ, s, s̞		s
w		w	

The alternation between [t], [d] does not appear to be contrastive in Kevin's speech, but instead shows great variation, e.g. *there* [tai], *that* [ɖæ], *fish* [tis], [ɖis]. There appears to be a tendency to change all apical stops to [t], with a phonetically varying [ɖ] appearing occasionally. The sound [s] also appears to be used contrastively with [t], but it shares phonetic variation, e.g. *fish* [tisθ], [tisˢ], *mouth* [naːsθ], *friends* ['entsʲ]. The [w] also shows phonetic variation: *was* [wɔz], *once* [wʌns], *little* [ɫʷitɫʷ]. The latter assumes a change of [l] → [w]. Haas notes that this [ɫʷ] is a labiovelar lateral ('dark' l) with rounding. Since this occurs only for [l] in the corpus, it may be that [w] [ɫʷ] are contrastive in Kevin's speech in pairs like *light*, *white*. If so, the phonemic inventory would need to be altered to show it. It would exemplify the use of a phonetic contrast not present in the adult language, although based upon the [l]–[w] adult distinction which is probably part of the child's perceptual system.

Here are some of the phonological processes that result in Kevin's phonemic inventory. The following affect fricatives.

$$
\begin{array}{llll}
\text{f} \rightarrow \text{t} & \eth \rightarrow \text{d} & \left\{\begin{array}{l}\theta \\ \text{s} \\ \text{š} \\ \text{z}\end{array}\right\} \rightarrow \text{s} & \begin{array}{ll}\textit{mouth} & [\text{naːs}] \\ \textit{fish} & [\text{tis}] \\ \textit{friends} & [\text{'ents}]\end{array} \\
\textit{fish} \quad [\text{tis}] & \textit{that} \quad [\text{dæ}]
\end{array}
$$

The [f] to [t] substitution also occurred in Ethel's speech. The substitutions into [s] show that stopping is being lost gradually. This is a common situation where a process is restricted until it is eventually lost. Fronting also occurs in the data, e.g. *good* [dud], *carpenter* [taːpentə]. There is even a case of the deletion of an initial unstressed syllable, *upon* [pan]. There are examples of other processes as well, but the shortage of materials does not allow an explicit analysis of any of the processes to be made. Overall, however, there is sufficient indication of the systematic use of phonological processes.

5.22   Tom, Jim and Frank

Despite the existence of both these studies, Compton (1970) provided the pioneer study in the demonstration of the systematic nature of deviant phonology. He did this while attempting to demonstrate the efficacy of using the principles of generative phonology. His subjects were Tom and Jim, two children with slightly above average intelligence and a speech defect that left their language 70 to 80 per cent unintelligible. He gave each the Templin–Darley and his own naming test, and wisely used three transcribers. After elaborate analyses of each, he concludes '[Jim's] pronunciation is also just as systematic and consistent as that of any other child or adult speaker of English whose speech is not deviant. This statement is, of course, just as true for Tom and the several other children we have studied, as well as for most other children with articulatory disorders' (336). Notice that deviant is used here in its general sense.

Ironically, while Compton's conclusion is valid, it is not at all clear that his analysis of the two boys' speech really reflects the phonological processes in use.

Unfortunately, it is nearly impossible to test his analysis since he does not give any examples of the children's words. Instead, he confines himself to tables of substitutions. Lorentz (1972) criticizes this, as well as the fact that Compton never considered the possible effect of environing sounds on substitutions. As will be shown, this can alter his analysis greatly.

Table 24 Twelve substitutions in Tom's speech as noted by Compton 1970

1	č → s	oblig.*		7	p → pᵏ	opt.
2	s → k	opt.		8	j → d	oblig.
3	f → k	oblig.		9	d → g	opt.
4	k → sk	opt.		10	z → s	oblig.
5	k → k⁼	opt.		11	š → s	opt.
6	t → t⁼	opt.		12	l → j	opt.

*oblig. = obligatory; opt. = optional.

The analysis of Tom's speech is confined to the production of initial consonants. Before an attempt is given to use generative theory to analyse Tom's speech, Compton lists the substitutions as twelve rules, as in table 24. Through the use of features, he reduces part of this list to three basic rules. Rather than attempt to describe his rule in features, which would take a lot of space, we can consider them in terms of the segments they affect.

Rule A: $\begin{Bmatrix} š \\ č \end{Bmatrix} \to s \qquad j \to d \qquad$ (Rules 1, 8, 11)

Rule B: $\quad s \to k$ (Rules 2, 9)
$\quad\quad\quad d \to g$

Rule C: $\begin{bmatrix} p \\ t \\ k \end{bmatrix} \to \begin{bmatrix} p^= \\ t^= \\ k^= \end{bmatrix} \qquad$ (Rules 5, 6, 7)

These three rules combine with rules 3, 4, 10, and 12 which are not changed.

In examining the child's system, one wants to find the most general rules possible. As important, however, is to find processes that are *natural processes* in language. For example, when a child makes a fricative into a stop this should demonstrate a general tendency in child language. Chapter 2 outlined a variety of natural processes that children follow. Looking at table 24, we can see some familiar ones. Both rules 10 and 12 are common, and 5, 6, 7 as revised in rule C reflect a general tendency in children to deaspirate stops. The latter was noted long ago in normal children by Jakobson (1968). Rules 3, 4 and 5, however, are unlike any process we have yet discussed. This suggests either that there is something unique about Tom's speech, or something wrong in Compton's analysis. The latter would be proved true if an alternative analysis of greater generality is possible which also is restricted to common processes of acquisition. This, in fact, can be done.

With regard to rule 4, Compton explains that this occurred as the result of Tom's clinician's attempt to correct his speech. Because of rule 2, Tom said [kak] for *sock*. To teach [s], the clinician had him say 'sssock'. The result was that Tom ended up saying 'ssskock' (325). This, then, can be traced to an artificial influence on his speech.

Next, notice that both rules 2 and 3 result in [k], i.e. [f] → [k]; [s] → [k]. The latter is combined by Compton with rule 9 in revised rule B. With reference to these rules, there is a similar process, the assimilation of alveolar stops to following velar ones, as discussed in chapter 2. Here some examples from Jennika's speech are repeated.

| *talk* | [kɔk] | *take* | [kek] | *duck* | [gʌk] |
| *dog* | [gɔk] | *Dick* | [gɪk] | *taco* | [kako] |

If assimilation is involved, then rules 2, 3 and 9 really involve two processes:

Stopping $\qquad \begin{Bmatrix} f \\ s \end{Bmatrix} \rightarrow t$

Assimilation $\qquad \begin{bmatrix} t \\ d \end{bmatrix} \rightarrow \begin{bmatrix} k \\ g \end{bmatrix} - V \begin{Bmatrix} k \\ g \end{Bmatrix}$

There are three pieces of information supporting this re-analysis. First, the stopping rule as now stated is a process we have seen already. Ethel had it, and Kevin had the first part of [f] → [t]. Secondly, there would need to be stimulus words with final [k]'s and [g]'s to cause the assimilation. Here are some words Compton used for testing: [f] *fork*, [s] *sock*, [č] *chicken*, and [d] *dog*. The stimulus list had several words with environments that would cause this assimilation. The list probably created a general tendency to use initial [k], even to the extent of putting it in a few forms where it normally would not occur. An interesting further piece of evidence in favour of this interpretation is that Tom did not show [f], [s], [š], [j] going to [k] or [g] when given the Templin–Darley test. This stands to reason, however, since the latter is not loaded with words with final [k]'s and [g]'s.

With these revisions, the rules in table 24 (or as revised with rules A, B, C) can now be stated as in table 25. These not only show the systematic nature of Tom's speech but also reflect common phonological processes.

Table 25   A revised set of rules for Tom's speech

i	Fronting:	$\begin{Bmatrix} č \\ š \end{Bmatrix} \rightarrow s$		(Rules 1,11)
ii	Stopping:	(a) f → t (oblig.)		(Rule 3)
		(b) s → t (opt.)		(Rule 2)
		(c) ǰ → d (oblig.)		(Rule 8)
iii	Assimilation:	$\begin{Bmatrix} t \\ d \end{Bmatrix} \rightarrow \begin{Bmatrix} k \\ g \end{Bmatrix} / - V \begin{Bmatrix} k \\ g \end{Bmatrix}$		(may be overgeneralized in test)
iv	Rule C			
v	Rules 4, 10, 12 as in Table 24			

Compton does not spend as much time on the analysis of Jim's speech as on Tom's. He does, however, highlight some of the most common characteristics. With regard to initial stops, the child shows the following substitutions:

Adult sound	Jim's substitution
/p–/	p or p$^=$
/b–/	b
/t–/	t or t$^=$; k
/d–/	d; g
/k–/	k or k$^=$; t
/g–/	g; d

Notice that deaspiration occurs with [p], [t], [k] just as with Tom. Next, there is a variation where [t], [d] sometimes become velars, and velar [k], [g], sometimes become alveolars [t], [d]. From this Compton concludes, 'some of Jim's errors, in contrast to Tom's, may be attributed to "faulty" discrimination. This is the case . . . for the initial alveolar and velar stops which show bidirectional confusion with each other . . . t ← → k, d ← → g' (332). When considering neighbouring sounds and general processes, however, a much simpler explanation is possible.

First, this variation does not occur with final stops. Thus, Compton would have to claim that only initial ones are not discriminated, a peculiar situation which would be difficult to justify. However, no justification is needed. What is occurring is probably the interaction of two processes:

$$\text{Fronting} \qquad \begin{bmatrix} k \\ g \end{bmatrix} \rightarrow \begin{bmatrix} t \\ d \end{bmatrix} / \# \!-\!$$

$$\text{Assimilation} \qquad \begin{bmatrix} t \\ d \end{bmatrix} \rightarrow \begin{bmatrix} k \\ g \end{bmatrix} / \!-\! V \begin{Bmatrix} k \\ g \end{Bmatrix}$$

Fronting was discussed in chapter 2, section 2.334 as a common tendency in children's speech. It was noted that some children will restrict it to any initial [k], [g], and not final ones. This appears to be what Jim has done. The occurrence of [t], [d] changing to [k], [g] can be explained by the velar assimilation, a process already discussed in Tom's speech, and one which Compton's list of words tends to elicit. Lastly, the fact that some initial [k], [g] occur for adult [k], [g] can be due to either of two causes: (1) optional use of fronting, or (2) occurrence of final [k] or [g] in the elicitation list. Since Compton does not give any data, it is impossible to decide between them.

The only other initial segment process provided for Jim's speech is that [m] either deletes or goes to [b], and [n] deletes. This requires two processes, one deleting nasals, optional for [b], and the other denasalization of [m] if the first does not occur. Denasalization of this kind has already been mentioned in chapter 2.

Compton then proceeds to give five general rules for the rest of Jim's errors. The first two deal with vowel and nasal consonant sequences. Vowels become nasal when followed by a nasal. This common assimilation process was discussed in section 2.334. Jim would also occasionally drop the nasal. The final three processes all deal with Jim's production of word final adult [m], [n], [ŋ]. The substitutes were:

adult	/–m/	/–n/	/–ŋ/	
	m	n		
child	mːp	nːt	ːk	in unstressed syllables
	mːp	nːtʻ	ːkʻ	
	mːb	nːd	ːg	in stressed syllables
	∅	∅		

Since final [m], [n], [ŋ] occurred, all three variations are optional. Rule 3 indicates that final nasals tend to become denasalized at the end of their production. This appears to be an intermediate step before denasalization is finally lost. In unstressed syllables, the segment also becomes devoiced. Rule 4 states that the voiced stops that are created are unusually long in some instances. Finally, rule 5 indicates that the voiceless stop may be heavily aspirated. Stating all these in segments, Tom's systematic processes are presented in table 26.

Table 26   The phonological processes, in segments, of Jim's speech

Initial consonants

i   Deaspiration: $\begin{bmatrix} p \\ t \\ k \end{bmatrix} \rightarrow \begin{bmatrix} p^= \\ t^= \\ k^= \end{bmatrix}$ / # — V   (opt.)

ii   Fronting: $\begin{bmatrix} k \\ g \end{bmatrix} \rightarrow \begin{bmatrix} t \\ d \end{bmatrix}$ / # — V

iii   Assimilation: $\begin{bmatrix} t \\ d \end{bmatrix} \rightarrow \begin{bmatrix} k \\ g \end{bmatrix}$ / — V $\begin{Bmatrix} k \\ g \end{Bmatrix}$

Vowels

iv   Nasalization: V → Ṽ / — $\begin{Bmatrix} m \\ n \\ ŋ \end{Bmatrix}$

Final consonants

v   Nasal deletion: [Nasal] → ∅ / — $\overset{C}{\#}$ (opt.)

vi   Denasalization: $\begin{bmatrix} m \\ n \\ ŋ \end{bmatrix} \rightarrow \begin{bmatrix} mb \\ nd \\ ŋg \end{bmatrix}$ / — #   (opt.)

vii   Devoicing: $\begin{bmatrix} mb \\ nd \\ ŋg \end{bmatrix} \rightarrow \begin{bmatrix} mp \\ mt \\ mk \end{bmatrix}$ / $\underset{\text{[-stress]}}{V}$ — #
i.e. in unstressed syllables

viii   Lengthening: $\begin{bmatrix} mb \\ nd \\ ŋg \end{bmatrix} \rightarrow \begin{bmatrix} mbː \\ ndː \\ ŋgː \end{bmatrix}$ / — #   (opt.)

ix   Aspiration: $\begin{bmatrix} mp \\ nt \\ ŋk \end{bmatrix} \rightarrow \begin{bmatrix} mpʻ \\ ntʻ \\ ŋkʻ \end{bmatrix}$ / — #   (opt.)

Before concluding the discussion of Compton's article, it is worth pointing out one further fact. While he succeeds in his argument to show that deviant phonology is systematic (although some of his rules require revision), it is not at all clear that he is equally successful in showing the need for a formal linguistic methodology. The formalism he uses is elaborate and difficult to follow; the statement of the processes in segments (as done above) rather than features is clearer and shows the same facts. Also, the formalism he uses is not even in current use in linguistic circles. It contains many errors and revisions on Compton's part that are never explained.

Recently, Compton (1975) has published another analysis of a deviant child. The child, referred to as Frank, was given Compton's list of words to be named.

This data was then analysed and used to construct a programme of therapy. Frank's phonology was then re-examined at six intervals to see how therapy altered his speech.

In this analysis, Compton has made some changes from his earlier approach. The rules are stated in segments rather than features, relaxing the strict use of a formal system. He also has begun to attempt to calculate percentages for the number of times a process occurs. Unfortunately he still does not consider the possibility of assimilations in the data, nor does he provide examples of the child's speech. Table 27 provides a revision of the 19 rules he provides, based on the approach we have been using. A few of the less striking processes have been omitted. Again, it is clear that the child's language is quite systematic. (This data will be returned to in the next chapter when we consider Compton's suggestions as to how therapy should proceed with this child's speech.)

Table 27 Some phonological processes of Frank's speech, as adapted from Compton 1975

Process		Compton's Rule No.
Assimilation: $\begin{bmatrix} t \\ d \end{bmatrix} \rightarrow \begin{bmatrix} k \\ g \end{bmatrix} / \_ V \begin{Bmatrix} k \\ g \end{Bmatrix}$		1
Affrication: $\begin{bmatrix} t \\ d \end{bmatrix} \rightarrow \begin{bmatrix} \check{c} \\ \check{j} \end{bmatrix} / \_ rV$		3
Fricative substitutions:		
Initial: $v \rightarrow w$ (50%)		4
$\begin{bmatrix} \theta \\ \eth \end{bmatrix} \rightarrow \begin{bmatrix} t \\ d \end{bmatrix} / \# \_$		5
$z \rightarrow s$		6
$s \rightarrow \check{s}$ (20%)		7
$\check{s} \rightarrow s$ (50%)		8
Final: $v \rightarrow f$ (50%)		15
$v \rightarrow b$ (50%)		
$\begin{bmatrix} \theta \\ \eth \end{bmatrix} \rightarrow \begin{bmatrix} s \\ z \end{bmatrix}$		18
$\begin{bmatrix} \check{c} \\ \check{j} \end{bmatrix} \rightarrow \begin{bmatrix} \check{s} \\ \check{z} \end{bmatrix} \rightarrow \begin{bmatrix} s \\ z \end{bmatrix}$		16, 17
$\begin{bmatrix} \check{s} \\ \check{z} \end{bmatrix} \rightarrow \begin{bmatrix} s \\ z \end{bmatrix}$		17
$z \rightarrow s$		19
Cluster reduction:		
$\begin{Bmatrix} r \\ l \end{Bmatrix} \rightarrow \emptyset / C \_ V$		9, 10
$s \rightarrow \emptyset / \_ C$		11
Liquid substitutions:		
$r \rightarrow w$		10
$l \rightarrow \begin{bmatrix} \emptyset \\ y \end{bmatrix}$ 60% 10%		9
Consonant devoicing:		
$\begin{bmatrix} b \\ d \\ g \end{bmatrix} \rightarrow \begin{bmatrix} p \\ t \\ k \end{bmatrix} / \_ \#$ (90%)		13

5.23 BN

The next study to appear demonstrating the systematic nature of deviant phonology was that of Pollock and Rees (1972).

> The child with the so-called 'functional' articulation disorder is more profitably viewed as a child with a linguistic disorder of a phonological type. This child's articulation pattern follows a consistent, regularized rule system. It is not the adult rule system, but an idiosyncratic set of rules that is nonetheless systematic. (453)

Here again the point is made that specific rules can be found in the child's speech. (The question of whether or not the rules are 'idiosyncratic' will be returned to in the next section.)

Pollock and Rees studied the development of three general phonological processes in the speech of a boy, B N, at each age: 5;2, 5;8, 6;3. The data shows not only the system of the child at one time, but also how it develops gradually, until acquisition is complete. This shows that the deviant child acquires phonology *gradually*, as does the normal child. It is not an all or nothing development.

The first process described is fronting. [k] was replaced by [t] and [j] by [d] at 5;2 and also at 5;8. In both periods it applied to initial segments. Finally, at 6;3 it was lost. The second process, dealing with the acquisition of [s], [z], [č], [j], was much more gradual. Here are the substitutions across the three periods.

Adult	5;2 Initial and final	5;8 Initial	Final	6;3 Initial	Final
/s/	s*	s*	s*	s*	s*
/č/	s*	č*	s	č*	s
/z/	z*	—	z*	—	z*
/j/	z	j*	z	j*	z

* denote correctness

These substitutions show two processes and two positions. The processes are:

(*1*) Loss of affrication: $\begin{bmatrix} č \\ j \end{bmatrix} \rightarrow \begin{bmatrix} š \\ ž \end{bmatrix}$

(*2*) Fronting: $\begin{bmatrix} š \\ ž \end{bmatrix} \rightarrow \begin{bmatrix} s \\ z \end{bmatrix}$

The two positions are initial and final.

At 5;2 both processes apply to all items. At 5;8 this has been limited by position. Both still apply to these sounds when at the end of the word. Initially, however, they no longer apply. Finally, at 6;3, the fronting process no longer occurs. (Note that it is also inapplicable for stops.) Loss of affrication still affects the final [č], and [j]. This demonstrates how processes are gradually lost.

These developments also show how elements are used contrastively in the child's speech. The contrasts at each age are:

5;3 Initial and final	5;8 Initial	Final	6;3 Initial	Final
s, z	s, z, č, š, j	s, z	s, z, č, š, j	s, z, š, ž

Just as processes gradually disappear, contrastive use gradually appears.

The third process is that of deletion of final consonants.

5;3	5;8	6;3
Deletion of all nasals, stops, fricatives	Stops are deleted $\begin{Bmatrix} t \\ d \end{Bmatrix} \to \emptyset$	p, k, b, d appear
	Nasals appear	Nasals occur
	$\begin{Bmatrix} f \\ v \end{Bmatrix} \to f$	f, v appear
	$\begin{Bmatrix} \theta \\ \eth \end{Bmatrix} \to d$	$\begin{bmatrix} \theta \\ \eth \end{bmatrix} \to \begin{bmatrix} t \\ d \end{bmatrix}$

At 5;3, all final consonants are deleted. Next, at 5;8, nasals are the first class of consonants to appear. This agrees with the data from Ethel, and the claims made by Renfrew (1966). Stops are deleted at 5;8, but the first attempts at fricatives begin. At 6;3 the stop consonants begin to occur with nasals although [t], [d] are omitted. The fact that [t], [d] occur as substitutes for [θ] and [ð] shows that it is not just a simple production problem. It is tied up with the general requirement of matching an adult model. Again, the child's development is shown as being both gradual and systematic.

5.24   Val, Jean, Vince, Jay and Curt

A more recent work on the systematic study of deviant phonology is Oller's (1973) paper 'Regularities in abnormal child phonology'. This study is actually a summary of a much longer unpublished paper by Oller *et al.* (1972) in which phonologies are written for five deviant children. Like Compton's work, these phonologies are done in a formal linguistic notation and are not backed up by examples from the child's speech. This is unfortunate in that the data could have been a valuable source of information. The unpublished paper does, however, have an appendix listing the rules for each child, thereby providing some ideas on the children's systems.

The five children studied were Val, Jean, Vince, Jay and Curt. In summarizing his analysis, Oller (1973) noted the following general findings:

(*1*)   All five children shared the process of reducing consonant clusters to one member: (*a*) [s] plus stop would reduce to stop; (*b*) stop plus liquid would reduce to stop; and (*c*) nasal plus consonants usually reduced to a consonant.

(*2*)   All five showed some processes affecting the production of fricatives: (*a*) the most common tendency was to either delete fricatives (especially for Vince in final position), or replace them with homorganic stops; (*b*) the labiodentals and interdental fricatives were often treated differently than other fricatives and affricates, the latter appearing to be the first acquired; (*c*) children treated fricatives differently depending on whether they were word initial or word final.

(*3*)   All children showed processes affecting liquids. Curt replaced them with stops; others changed them to more vowel-like elements ([o], [ə], [w]) depending on the position in the word. (The latter reflects the two processes referred to in this book as vocalization and gliding.) Oller concludes that all these reflect regular patterns of the phonology of these children.

Oller 1973 concludes with an example from Curt's speech to show systematicity. Curt made what appeared to be a random use of the stops [b], [d]. A closer examination of his speech, however, revealed that [b] occurred before low vowels and [d] before non-low vowels, e.g. *baby* [dɪdɪ], *dog* [baː]. Oller notes, 'it is clear that Curt's treatment of consonants was not totally random; indeed his treatment was extremely systematic' (46).

Since Curt's speech was the most reduced of the five subjects, and most subject to a claim of being unsystematic, it is useful to see how systematic it really was. Table 28 provides a revised set of the rules for Curt's speech as given in Oller *et al* 1972. In discussion of his sample, which was highly unintelligible, they say: 'our first impressions were that his speech was near random. This impression turned out to be quite incorrect. We found that with a very complex set of rules it was possible to capture some fascinating generalities with respect to his substitutions' (29).

Table 28   A restatement of Curt's phonology, based on data given in Oller *et al.* 1972)

1 Vowel neutralization: $V \rightarrow a / \_\_ \begin{Bmatrix} nasal \\ liquid \end{Bmatrix}$ (opt.)

$\begin{Bmatrix} ɔ \\ æ \\ ʌ \end{Bmatrix} \rightarrow a \qquad \begin{Bmatrix} i \\ ɪ \\ e \\ ɛ \\ o \\ u \end{Bmatrix} \rightarrow i$

2 Consonant replacement: All consonants $\rightarrow$ b / $\_\_$ Vowel

3 Consonant reduplication: $\begin{matrix} \#, V, C \ V \\ 1 \quad 2 \quad 3 \ 4 \end{matrix} \Rightarrow \begin{matrix} \#C \ VC \ V \\ 13 \quad 23 \ 4 \end{matrix}$

4 Height assimilation: b $\rightarrow$ d / $\_\_$ i

5 Regressive vowel assimilation: $\breve{V} \rightarrow \begin{bmatrix} a \\ i \end{bmatrix} / \begin{bmatrix} a \\ i \end{bmatrix} C \_\_$

i.e. unstressed vowels assimilate to preceding vowel

6 Vowel lengthening: V $\rightarrow$ V: / $\_\_$ Voiced consonant

7 Final consonant deletion: (a) C $\rightarrow$ Ø / $\_\_$ #   (opt.)
except final fricatives
(b) C $\rightarrow$? / $\_\_$ #

8 Fricative metathesis: $\begin{matrix} \# \begin{Bmatrix} s \\ š \end{Bmatrix} V(C) \qquad \#(C)V \begin{Bmatrix} s \\ š \end{Bmatrix} \\ 1 \quad 2 \quad 3 \ 4 \Rightarrow 1 \ 4 \quad 3 \ 2 \end{matrix}$

9 Fricative substitution: Fricative $\rightarrow$ č / $\_\_$ #

10 h deletion: h $\rightarrow$ Ø / # $\_\_$

11 Reduction of clusters: (a) Stop $\rightarrow$ Ø / #s $\_\_$
(b) $\begin{Bmatrix} r \\ l \end{Bmatrix} \rightarrow$ Ø / when next to consonant
(c) Nasal $\rightarrow$ Ø / when next to stop

Several of the processes are similar to those in chapter 2 for reduced phonologies. Vowel neutralization results in a basic two vowel system. The use oʿ two initial consonants [b], [d], with an alternation based on the quality of the vowel was noted by Jakobson (*cf.* table 13 and the discussion thereon). Other processes discussed there are 5, 6, 7 and 10. Process 3 reflects the basic CVCV structure that children tend to preserve. Examples of its application are *airplane* [dɪdɪ]; *apple* [baba]. The processes 6, 7, 8, and 9 all reflect the fact that Curt has a perceptual schema for words with the shape (C)Vč. Examples that lead to these rules are: *sock, saw* [æč]; *ship* [dɪč]; *leaf, goose, vase* [ʌːč]. Examples of processes 6 and 7 are *car, dog* [baː]; *cat, duck* [ba] or [baʔ]; *chair* [baː] or [dɪː]; *rake, jeep* [dɨʔ]. The reduction of clusters is typical of other children except that [s] is retained instead of the stop. This is not well documented so little can be said about it. It is an example of what was called the deletion of the unmarked member in chapter 2. The analysis of Curt's speech by Oller *et al.* provides an excellent example of how system can be found in very unintelligible child speech.

5.25 Bernie, Marc, Jennifer and Christina

Currently the richest source of information on the nature of deviant phonology is the excellent study by Edwards and Bernhardt (1973a). Trained in doing fine phonetic transcriptions of children's speech, the authors collected and analysed elicited words from four children, Bernie 3;3, Marc 3;3, Jennifer 4;4 and Christina 5;3. They are not concerned with formalism but with the identification of phonological processes, and give several examples from the children's speech of each process discussed. Their analyses are the most detailed ever presented on this topic.

The first child, Bernie is the most intelligible of the four. His speech appears to be very systematic. Marc is next in intelligibility. 'Marc's speech is sometimes unintelligible. Analysis reveals that he tends to make somewhat inconsistent substitutions, but that the substitutions *are* in fact consistent within a certain range of variation' (14). Christina is the least intelligible of the children, with several simplifying processes. Jennifer, the next to least in intelligibility, reveals a less systematic phonology than the other three. 'Much of Jennifer's speech is mumbled, and there are many inconsistencies in her speech . . . the result is the postulation of many optional processes, often with several exceptions or idiosyncratic items. In short, her phonological "system" is not as systematic as it is for most children, even those with language problems' (22). This is the first real case of a child with a marginally systematic phonology and it is worth examining more closely later.

After examining each child's phonology in detail, Edwards and Bernhardt compare those processes shared by at least two children. Table 29 presents those processes shared in varying degrees by each child.

Table 29 Processes shown by Bernie, Marc, Jennifer and Christina, from Edwards and Bernhardt 1973

1 The reduction of consonant clusters (B, M, J, C)
    (a) Loss of *s*
    (b) Reduction of Nasal + Stop to one member
2 Stopping of fricatives and affricates (B, M, J, C)
3 Labial assimilation (B, M, J, C)
4 Labialization of obstruents in clusters (B, M, J, C)
5 Voicing changes (B, M, J, C)
    (a) Voicing of consonants before vowels
    (b) Devoicing of final consonants
6 Fronting
    (a) Palatals (B, M, J, C)
    (b) Velars (M, C)
7 Loss of final consonants (M, J)
8 Neutralization of labials (M, J)
9 Nasal intrusion (J, C)
10 Velar assimilation (J, C)
11 Nasal assimilation (J, C)
12 Metathesis (J, C)

The first six processes occur in one form or another for all the children. One and two are common ones that we have seen in the other children discussed so far. The third, labial assimilation, is shared by all, but does not appear frequently. (The transcriptions here are simplified from the fine phonetic ones in their paper.)

Bernie—initial voiced continuants are labialized—no examples

Marc—	*knife*	[wap]	*Jennifer*—*zebra*	[wɪpʷʌ]
	number	[wambə]	*TV*	[fwɪpʊɪ]
	mommy	[wɔmɛ]	*table*	[bɛbɪ]

The labialization of obstruents in clusters is a process discussed for normal children in chapter 2. None of the previous analyses really isolated this process in the deviant children, but the data here suggest that it may be common. Some examples are:

Bernie		*Marc*		*Jennifer*		*Christina*	
three	[pʰɪ]	*truck*	[baʔ]	*clown*	[fʷan]	*three*	[fwə]
swing	[fwɛŋ]	*clown*	[pẇa]	*green*	[fwɪn]		
		three	[pʷɪi]	*glove*	[fᶷɔːʔ]		
		dress	[bas]	*glasses*	[fˡæsɪ]		

Like the above process, voicing processes have not been a striking feature of previous analyses, with the exception of Frank's speech which showed final devoicing. Here, they appear to be part of each child's phonology. Processes 6, 7 and 10 have been common in previous data. The eighth one listed, neutralization of labials, is a process that occurs in both Marc's and Jennifer's sample. It is a tendency to replace labial consonants (the result of assimilation in some cases) with the glide [w]. Some examples are:

Marc		*Jennifer*	
fish	[wæʔ]	*bottle*	[wado]
teddybear	[tɛwʌ]	*fork*	[wʊk]
knife	[wap]	*face*	[wɛɪ]
mommy	[wɔmɛ]	*vase*	[wɛns]
number	[wambə]	*bath*	[wæf]

The last three processes for discussion, 8, 11 and 12 are all shared by the two least intelligible children, Jennifer and Christina. This suggests that these may be more basic processes of reduced speech. Earlier data of Ethel and Jim show a tendency to have nasal and consonant sequences. Jennifer and Christina have a process of nasal intrusion. This occurs at syllable boundaries for Christina (like Ethel) and at the end of words for Jennifer (as with Jim).

Jennifer		*Christina*	
bridge	[pfwɪnt]	*station*	[tʰentʰɪn]
red	[wænt]	*Christine*	[tʰəntɪn]
bird	[bɽⁿd]		

Nasal assimilation results in a consonant assimilating to a noncontiguous nasal, e.g. Jennifer—*jamas* [namɛs], *candle* [nʌno]; Christina—*magazine* [mənotɪn]; *elephant* [anafɪn]. Metathesis accounts for a few peculiar forms that apparently result from interchanging consonants, Jennifer—*pencil* [pɛsnə]; Christina—*fish* [sɪp], [twʊf], [čɪp], [šɪp]. Of the less common processes, like the latter ones, there are few examples. Overall, however, there is sufficient data to demonstrate the systematic use of phonological processes.

Table 30 Some general processes and exceptions to them in Jennifer's speech

Process		Examples		Exceptions	
1	Cluster reduction:	*spoon*	[pʊ]	*spoon*	ʈfʊ]
	loss of s	*snoopy*	[nʊpɪ]	*snoopy*	[snʊpi]
		stockings	[tʌkɪns]	*stuck*	[sʌk]
2	Loss of final consonants	*leaf*	[nɪi]	*knife*	[nʌs]
		mouth	[mæᵘ]	*bath*	[wæf]
		face	[weˡ]	*juice*	[dus]
		fish	[pfʌ]	*brush*	[wʌɵ]
3	Cluster reduction:	*lamp*	[nɛm]	*pumpkin*	[pʊgæn]
	nasal + stop	*hand*	[hɛɪn]	*orange*	[oᵘʊnt]
		candle	[kʰæno]	*pink*	[pʰɪŋk]

Since the authors consider Jennifer's phonology to be less systematic than the others, it is important to examine this claim closely. The list of processes demonstrates that she has many processes in common with the other children. Her use of them, however, varies. Whereas the other children show a tendency either to apply a process or not, Jennifer's usage fluctuates a great deal. It is almost as if she decides at random whether to apply them or not. As a result, there are numerous examples of exceptions to most of her general processes. Table 30 provides some of these. This suggests that the systematic aspects of the child's phonology may show wider ranges of variation than the normal child's. This anticipates the discussion of this question in the next section.

5.26 Joe and David

The last two children to be discussed were both studied by Lorentz. Like Jennifer's speech, their language presents properties that raise the question of what constitutes deviance, which is discussed in the next section. Both show systematic phonologies, but phonologies that do not look like those of the younger normal child.

The first child, Joe, is reported on in Lorentz (1972). Joe has a very well-developed phonological system, except for his treatment of certain specific consonant clusters in English. (He also substitutes [f] for [θ] and [b] for [v] but these are normal for this age and will not be included in the discussion.) His speech is clear and shows these patterns consistently. They are given in table 31 together with examples of each.

Table 31   Joe's substitution patterns for specific clusters, examples and the rule that produce them, adapted from Lorentz 1972

Adult cluster	Child's substitute	Examples			
1 sw	f	swoop	[f]oop;	swat	[f]at
	(or) fw	swim	[fw]im;	swing	[fw]ing
2 sm	f Ṽ	smoke	[fõwk];	small	[fãl]
3 sp	f	spoon	[f]oon;	spot	[f]ot
4 sn	s Ṽ	snap	[sæp];	snake	[sẽyk]
5 st	s	story	[s]ory;	stand	[s]and
6 sk	ks	scan	[ks]ar;	scout	[ks]out

Rules

A   Labial assimilation to obstruent $s \rightarrow f / \_ \begin{Bmatrix} p \\ m \\ w \end{Bmatrix}$

B   Vowel nasalization: $V \rightarrow \tilde{V} \ /C \begin{Bmatrix} m \\ n \end{Bmatrix} \_$

C   Metathesis: $\underset{1}{s}, \underset{2}{k}, \underset{3}{V} \rightarrow \underset{2}{k}, \underset{1}{s}, \underset{3}{V}$

D   Cluster reduction (of unmarked member):

(1) $\begin{Bmatrix} m \\ n \\ t \end{Bmatrix} \rightarrow \emptyset / s \_ V$

(2) $w \rightarrow \emptyset / s \_ V$ (opt.)

These show a small set of rules persisting in the child's speech. We have not yet seen cases of rules like B and C. With regard to D, it is a case of the unmarked member of the cluster being deleted. With normal children, this does not occur frequently. With Joe, not only does it occur, but is used in all cases in his speech. That is, it is a very strong process. This suggests that not only is Joe's speech systematic, but also different from the normal child's.

The other child studied by Lorentz is David, a four-year-old with a much more severely affected phonology than Joe. Lorentz (1974) says that David's speech was almost completely unintelligible, and that only vowels and nasals were pronounced without being affected by a simplification process of some kind. All were used in a systematic fashion, although several were unlike anything discussed so far.

As for more usual processes, there were several that have already been seen in one form or another. Fronting occurred for [t] and [k], e.g. *duck* [dət], *dog* [dad]. Medially, stops were occasionally deleted or else replaced by a glottal stop, e.g. *pretty* [plɪtiy], *daughter* [dɔɾ], *kitten* [kiʔɪn]. Final fricatives were deleted, e.g. *bees* [biy]; *teeth* [tiy]; *love* [lə], *this* [dɪʰ]. Somewhat more unusual was David's treatment of nasal + stop sequences. Regardless of the voicing of the stop, the nasal is retained, e.g. *pins* [pɪn], *hand* [æn], *pink* [pɪŋ], *ink* [ɪːŋ].

His treatment of certain fricatives and glides was even more unusual. For some fricatives, David used stopping as expected; [v] went to [b] and [ð] to [d]. Even the substitution of [w] for [f] is not too unusual, and was also done by Smith's (1973) son A. For the rest, however, the following pattern emerged (55).

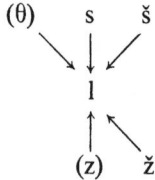

That is, they all become lateral [l].

sing	[lɪŋ]	*shell*	[læl]	*thing*	[lɪŋ]
such	[lət]	*sharp*	[larp]	*think*	[liyː]
so	[low]	*sheep*	[liyp]	but *thumb*	[wəm]

This is a very uncommon pattern of substitution.

The liquid /r/ altered between correct use and a [w]. Like David's pattern for labiodentals, this is an expected process, e.g *run* [wən], [rən]. In clusters, however, all consonant plus [w] sequences (whether adult [w] or the substitute for /r/) showed liquid substitution.

pretty	[plɪtiy]	*twelve*	[tlɛl]
brother	[blə ʔɾ]	*twinkle*	[tlɪŋ ʔow]
true	[tluw]	*queen*	[kliyn]

This preference for the lateral also occurred as a substitution for /y/.

yes	[lɛʰ]	*your*	[lɾ]
you	[luw]	*yellow*	[lɛl]

David's speech shows a systematic use of both common and uncommon processes. It demonstrates that the issue of systematicity is just one aspect of deviant phonology that needs to be considered. Even if deviant speech is systematic, the next question is whether this system is like that of the younger normal child, or whether it is unique in distinctive ways.

5.3   Do deviant children have deviant systems?

While the previous section demonstrated that the deviant child's speech is very systematic, it took no position with regard to whether or not this system is more or less the same as that of the younger normal child. The comparison with normal acquisition cannot be made in one step. There are several ways that the deviant child's system may differ from the normal's. These are in the nature of phonological processes, the use of phonological processes, their order of appearance, and the use of sounds as contrastive elements. There are at least three positions that one could take on this issue:

(1)   The deviant child shows *delayed* acquisition, his system is much the same as a younger normal child.
(2)   The deviant child has the same phonological processes as the normal, but uses them in a different way. Certain processes then tend to persist longer than

they would in the normal child. In this sense the resulting system is *different* from the normal child's although the processes are the same.

(*3*)   The deviant child shows some processes that are similar to the normals, but others that are unique to deviant children. The child also persists in using certain processes longer than the normal child.

Delay	*Deviance 1*	*Deviance 2*
same processes;	same processes;	unique processes;
same general use	persistent use	persistent use

As will be seen, the second position has been the dominant one in the literature.

5.31   Types of phonological processes in deviant phonology

A comparison of the processes proposed for the children discussed in this chapter with those mentioned for normal children shows a striking number of similarities. Children show a tendency to reduce clusters, delete final consonants, make fricatives into stops, change liquids into glides etc. Several studies have noted this similarity. Oller (1973), for example, states 'it should be clear that the rules are apparently not unlike those of normal child phonology. Even the rules which are not held by all five subjects show remarkable similarity to normal child processes' (44). This same observation was also made by Edwards and Bernhardt (1973a): 'Although the children discussed in this paper have been called unintelligible, it is striking that the individual phonological processes underlying their substitutions are, for the most part, quite normal' (48). Table 32 shows the distribution of the most common phonological processes discussed in the various studies of 17 deviant children.

Table 32   The occurrence of the most common phonological processes among 17 deviant children (cf. table 23)

Process	*Ethel*	*Kevin*	*Tom*	*Jim*	*Frank*	*BN*	*Val*	*Jean*	*Vince*	*Jay*	*Curt*	*Bernie*	*Marc*	*Jennifer*	*Christina*	*Joe*	*David*
Cluster reduction	×	×			×		×	×	×	×	×	×	×	×	×	×	
Stopping	×	×			×		×	×	×	×	×	×	×	×			
Depalatalization	×	×	×		×	×		×	×	×		×	×	×	×		
Fronting	×	×	×	×	×	×			×	×	×		×		×		×
Gliding	×	×	×		×		×	×	×			×	×	×	×		
Deletion of final C	×			×		×			×		×		×	×	×		×
Voicing processes			×	×							×	×	×	×	×		
Assimilation in clusters				×								×	×	×	×	×	
Velar assimilation		×	×	×									×	×			

× indicates at least some use of the process

Although this table shows that deviant children show by and large the same processes, there is still some evidence that deviant children also use some processes that are unusual by normal standards. The exact specification of the variety and limits of these requires a great deal of future research. The data provided on the 17 deviant children, however, provides enough examples to make an initial examination.

In looking at unusual processes, there are two possible interpretations of their nature. One is that they are the *common use of uncommon processes*; that is the process is one that normal children may show, but never for very long. For example, it is much more common for the normal child to delete the marked member of a consonant cluster than the unmarked. He will, however, show the reverse occasionally. The deviant child who deletes the unmarked member throughout cannot be said to be using a unique process, but rather one that normal children use. The deviant child's widespread use of this process suggests that it has a more fundamental role in his system. The second possibility is that deviant children occasionally use *unique processes*, ones that normal children never show. In the following discussion there will be no attempt to deal separately with each type, although some comments will be made when relevant. A clear separation will not be possible until we know with certainty what the normal processes are.

The following are examples of unusual phonological processes in the speech of deviant children:

(*1*) In Ethel's speech, there was the occasional use of *lisping*, i.e. the use of [θ]. While normal children show some distortion of [s] for several years (*cf.* Ingram 1975a), the distinct use of a lisp has been a classic disorder of speech.

(*2*) Ethel, Kevin and Tom all showed the substitution of [t] for [f]. (This could be called *tetism*, i.e. the substitute of t, in the sense of Panagos, 1974). Data from normal children, however, suggests that [f] is acquired very early (*cf.* Ingram 1975a). When normal children do substitute for [f], it is usually by stopping to [p] or gliding to [w].

(*3*) Three deviant children showed the use of a lateral for [s]. David used a voiced [l], as shown in the previous section. Pollack and Rees referred to a four-year-old boy who used a voiceless lateral fricative for [s] (453). Lastly, another study by Edwards and Bernhardt (1973b) refers to a boy John (age 5;2) who used a voiced lateral fricative for [s]. This is not usually found in normal children.

(*4*) Several of the children tended to use nasalization where it usually would not be expected. This could be referred to as *nasal preference*. Ethel showed the rule of [w] → [m], which was later adjusted to ∅ → m / # __ Consonant. This was a tendency to place an [m] at the beginning of words. Both Bernie and Jennifer showed a similar process. With regard to Bernie, Edwards and Bernhardt state 'the only exceptional process concerns the change of initial /w/ . . . to bilabial nasal [m]. Sometimes /w/ is correct, but just as frequently [m] is substituted . . . similarly, a [w] resulting from /r/ . . . may change to an [m]' (6). An example is *rabbit* [mavɛ ?]. Jennifer did not show the above change of [w] to [m] but did substitute [n] for [l]. 'Nasals are important sounds for Jennifer. . . . Nasals are often retained in her speech at the expense of other sounds' (22). Lastly, Christina changed all word final alveolar and palatal fricatives and affricates into a 'voiceless nasal snort' (36).

(*5*) Several of the children showed a *fricative preference*, i.e. a tendency to retain and/or move fricatives and affricates. Some children showed metathesis. Curt deleted final segments in general but metathesized fricatives to final position and kept them, e.g. *sock* [æč]; *ship, leaf, goose* [dič]. Christina showed metathesis in the other direction, e.g. *fish* [sɪp], [šɪp], [čɪp]. A boy I observed, Aaron, also did this, e.g. *desk* [sək], *basket* [səkə]. Jay occasionally changed some final stops to [č] and [s], although no examples are given. Another way to show fricative preference is to retain [s] in clusters. Both Jay and Joe showed this.

(6) While reduplication is a common process in young normal children, there is still no well documented case of its use by a deviant child.

One pattern that appears in these isolated cases is a tendency to overuse some articulation that has been developed. It suggests that the child tries to compensate for difficulties by using an element with which he feels familiar. More research into the entire question of deviant patterns, however, is required.

5.32 The use of phonological processes

The impression of several investigators has been that the deviant child differs not so much by the nature of the processes as by the way that they persist in the child's system. The normal child presumably uses processes to simplify speech in some relatively consistent order. This was hinted at in chapter 2 when it was noted, for example, that the deletion of final consonants begins to disappear around the appearance of the fiftieth word. For the deviant child, however, these processes may persist and subsequently occur side-by-side with other processes with which they normally would not coincide.

Edwards and Bernhardt describe this very nicely in the discussion of their results.

> The phonologies written for these children are not entirely similar to those for 'normal' children, even those who are much younger. Normal children who exhibit processes like prevocalic voicing generally do so at a stage before they have two and three syllable words. The children in this study have multisyllabic words, and yet they still have the rather infertile process of prevocalic voicing. There are several such examples where processes common in young children are found along with processes characteristic of older children. (48)

While the support for this needs a firmer understanding of the order of development of phonological patterns in normal children, this provides a substantial hypothesis on the nature of deviance.

An example of evidence in favour of this hypothesis is the article by Renfrew (1966), 'Persistence of the open syllable in defective articulation'. She has noted that there are certain children with phonological disability who show a persistent use of the deletion of final consonants, thereby maintaining an open CV syllable structure. The normal child will have acquired only a few initial consonants before final ones begin to be used. Children with the persistent deletion of final consonants, however, will acquire most initial consonants before using any finally.

This position of deviant systems resulting from the persistence of some processes is also argued for by Lorentz (1972). He states that the rules do not disappear when expected, but persist in the system, eventually affecting other processes. As a result, he says: 'It is unlikely that any typically complex deviant phonological system would be equivalent in all respects to any normal stage of phonological development' (7). Joe is given as an example of such a situation. Compton (1975) expresses a similar position.

While table 32 indicates that certain processes are common for deviant children, it is also apparent that deviant children will vary as to which processes will persist in their speech. That is, different children will have different combinations of the processes that are still operating in their language. This can be exemplified by the four subjects observed by Edwards and Bernhardt (1973a) in two processes—the deletion of final consonants, and the fronting of velar consonants.

	Bernie	Marc	Jennifer	Christina
Final consonant deletion	no	yes	no	yes
Fronting	no	yes	yes	no

Bernie showed neither process, and Marc had both. The girls showed one each. This kind of variation was found by Weber (1970) in a comparison of the persistent processes shown by 18 children with moderate to severe disorders. Table 32 does not provide a convincing spread of processes since the children described were observed by different investigators with different analytic interests. In Weber's study, all 18 subjects received the Templin–Darley test and were analysed by him. Table 33 displays the use of various patterns across his subjects. As can be seen, they varied with regard to which processes persisted in their speech. Subject C, for example, showed only stopping, whereas others showed several processes.

Table 33   The occurrence of phonological patterns in 18 children studied by Weber 1970

Processes	A	B	C	D	E	F	G	H	I	J	K	L	M	N	O	P	Q	R
Fronting of velars	×				×			×					×				×	
Fronting of palatals	×	×		×	×		×	×	×	×	×	×			×	×	×	
Loss of affrication		×				×	×								×			
Stopping			×								×	×	×		×			×
Gliding							×	×			×	×		×			×	
Affrication								×		×							×	
Devoicing										×					×			
Final consonant deletion												×		×				
Other			×		×			×				×	×		×			

In comparing tables 32 and 33, we see that the processes of forward articulation (fronting of velars and fronting of palatals) and of stopping are both widespread. The question could be posed whether these occur more with deviant children than with younger normal children. Menyuk (1968) found some evidence to support this. In a distinctive feature analysis of normal and deviant children, she found three features lacking overall in the deviant group. These were [+strident], [−anterior] and [+continuant]. The first and third would be eliminated by stopping, and the second by fronting.

Besides drawing the conclusion that processes persist in deviant speech, Edwards and Bernhardt proceed to make the following additional conclusion: 'The main difference between the children in this study and normal children appears to be that these children exhibit *more* phonological processes and less consistent processes. This is what makes them unintelligible' (48). That is, not only do processes persist, but the deviant child will not match the younger normal child because he shows more simplifying processes than the latter. Adding to the variation is the fact that the processes will also fluctuate more for the deviant child. The latter is particularly exhibited in the speech of Jennifer.

The conclusion about variation fits their data but contrasts with what Lorentz has claimed on this issue:

> Another important difference between developing phonologies and typical deviant systems is the small amount of variation to be found in such deviant systems. That is, aberrant phonological systems of four and five year old children are relatively fixed and consistent in terms of the operations of the rules of that system. (8)

How can opposing views like this be reconciled?

A partial answer on the issue of variation appears to reside in the severity of the disorder. The children observed by Edwards and Bernhardt were highly unintelligible. Joe, on the other hand, had fairly clear speech and only a limited set of processes. Consequently, Lorentz's point may be true only for children with limited problems of the kind shown by Joe.

With regard to the claim that deviant children have more processes, this can only be decided through comparative studies with normal children. At the moment it remains a possible but not proven hypothesis.

5.33   The use of contrast

There is one further way in which one can examine how the deviant child's speech may differ from that of the normal. This concerns children's use of sounds to contrast meanings. As discussed in chapter 2, a major task of the child's acquisition of language is to keep the form of different words separate. For example, if the child is trying to say the words *food* and *foot*, he needs to show in his speech that these are separate words. One way is to simply say them as the adult does. The young child, however, cannot always do this. Suppose that the child in our example has a process of devoicing final consonants, as well as one that substitutes [u] for [ʊ]. The two words would both be pronounced [fut]. That is, they would be *homonyms*. To avoid this, the child has an alternative. This is the use of some aspect of the child's own sound system to show the difference. In this example, the child could use vowel length and say [fuːt] and [fut] respectively. It was in reference to the use of sounds in this fashion that the organizational level was described. The contrastive use of vowel length was part of Joan Velten's phonology (Velten 1943).

Since young children have several simplifying processes, one would expect that they would have many homonyms. In a recent study, however, this did not prove to be the case (*cf.* Ingram 1975c). After examining five children's spontaneous language at approximately age 1;6, I found there were surprisingly few homonyms. It appeared that the children were quite good at keeping their words distinct, even if not pronouncing them with correct adult form. The methods for doing this varied. Some simply did not seem to have homonyms. Others did, but used alternate pronunciations for one or both. A third method was to change one of the words by a unique phonological process. For example, my daughter Jennika had correct production of word initial [m] and [n]. The word for *milk*, however, was [nʌk]. This should have been [mʌk] by the rules of her system. The latter, however, was used for the name of a neighbourhood friend *Mark*. The unique use of [n] for [m] allowed her to avoid the homonyms. It allowed the names to be contrasted.

If further evidence confirms this tendency in normal children, the question arises whether or not deviant children do this. The data from Jennifer suggest not. Her rules showed a great deal of inconsistency. This would mean that pronunciations often varied, and probably that there was not consistent use of contrasts. Also, her use of several simplifying processes suggests the creation of homonymy.

While this is largely a hypothesis, requiring close study, I can present some data to reflect the kind of situation that results from not keeping words distinct. Below are some examples of homonyms in Aaron's speech.

> *butter, ladder, letter, spider, water, whistle* [dado]
> *cup, foot, top* [pat]
> *belt, boat* [tap]
> *bear, pear* [peo]

The form [dado] is used for six different words. This results in a low level of intelligibility. One of the reasons that young normal children do so well communicating with their parents is the avoidance of multiple homonyms like this. If deviant children do not use contrasts to keep words separate, this will result in unintelligibility. This indicates that not only do contrasts need to be taught to these children, but also that forms like [dado] would be the first candidates. (This will be returned to in chapter 6.)

5.34 Summary

It appears that the deviant child has a deviant system, but care needs to be taken in defining the latter. The phonological processes that the deviant child draws upon are by and large the same as those used by the normal child to simplify speech. At the same time, there are some indications that the deviant child may also use either unique processes not found in normal speech or uncommon processes in a much more general fashion. The more striking aspect of the deviant system is that the processes do not always drop out in the normal order, but instead persist in the system. This results in a system where very early processes coexist with later ones. Individual children will vary with regard to which processes persist, although certain ones (e.g. fronting, stopping, gliding, cluster reduction, deletion of final consonants) appear more likely than others. In the system of the highly unintelligible child, these processes may be very inconsistent, resulting in a great deal of variation in pronunciation of the same word. In the less severe cases, on the other hand, there may be only a few well-established processes that are quite consistent in use.

Two further aspects may also characterize the deviant system, although they require further investigation. One is that the deviant child may use more processes than the younger normal child at a similar stage. The other is that the deviant child may not be as effective in using sounds contrastively as the normal child.

5.4   Types of phonological disorders

The kinds of issues discussed so far can be related to each specific type of phonological disorder. It is certainly possible that specific disorders will each have its own specific characteristics. This section will highlight some of the findings available on the phonological characteristics of specific types of phonological disorder.

5.41   Redefining 'functional articulation disorders'

Most of the children dealt with above would come under the category of functional articulation disorders. That is, there is no noticeable organic reason for their speech being abnormal. For example, Oller (1973) refers to his subjects as 'Five children . . . whose articulation appeared to be delayed in development. The subjects were otherwise basically normal' (37). For Tom and Jim, Compton (1970) reported: 'Each had a slightly above average IQ . . . and neither showed evidence of hearing loss or any physical anomalies which would cause his speech to be abnormal' (316).

Recently, efforts have been made to redefine this kind of disorder in linguistic terms. In chapter 2 a distinction was made between a child's organizational and production abilities. The former is concerned with being able to establish contrasts in language, i.e. to establish a system, whereas the latter is concerned with actually producing the sounds. These two can also be referred to as *phonemic* and *phonetic* abilities respectively. Recent papers have emphasized the need to distinguish these two in discussing a child's errors (*cf.* Moskowitz, 1972, Pollock and Rees 1972, Oller 1973). Pollock and Rees point out the difference between these two types of errors. 'The speech of the child who makes phonemic errors, predominantly, reflects his inadequate or deviant phonological system rather than his ability to plan or execute selected articulatory movements' (453). They then conclude that children with functional articulation disorders show phonemic rather than phonetic errors. In doing so, they suggest that we need a linguistic typology. 'This child has been traditionally classified as suffering from a 'functional' articulation disorder, although this term is empty and meaningless. The child with the so-called 'functional' articulation disorder is more profitably viewed as a child with a linguistic disorder of a phonological type' (453).

This difference has been demonstrated by pointing out that these children may not produce a sound correctly, and yet use that sound as a substitute for another one. For example, Oller (1973, 45) notes that Jean would make [š] into [t]. At the same time, however, she would substitute [š] for [č]. The production of [š], then, was not determined by articulatory factors, but also by the overall nature of her linguistic system. This is typical of normal children and shows that acquisition is more than just the production of sounds.

If this disorder is redefined as a linguistic one, the question also can be raised whether or not one can talk of phonological disability independently of other linguistic systems such as morphology, syntax, and semantics. Shriner, *et al.* (1969) report on research that has indicated that children with articulating defects also show more limited syntax than similar children without speech defects. Shriner *et al.* (1970) refer to this as the 'synergistic aspect' of language, that is, that it is a complex interlocking system. Panagos (1974) has recently argued that the use of open syllables actually reflects a more 'global' deficit in the child, reflecting grammatical and cognitive problems. Evidence reflecting deficits in areas other than just phonology is also found in Whitacre *et al.* 1970 and Menyuk and Looney 1972. Panagos, in his discussion, concludes, '. . . severe articulation disorders . . . should be incorporated into the clinical categorization *phonological disorder*, technically referring to restrictions in knowledge and use of phonological rules. . . . The presence of deviations of the sound system, furthermore, should be regarded as greatly increasing the probability of deficits of the syntactic and semantic components as well' (30). Evidence like this suggests that deviant phonology may be not just a phonemic disorder, but a more global linguistic one. As will be discussed in chapter 6, this added dimension provides some important implications for therapy.

5.42   Mental retardation

Studies on the articulation of mentally retarded children include those of Irwin 1942, Bangs 1942, Karlin and Strazzula 1952 and Schlanger 1953a and b. In general, each indicates that retarded children show similar substitution patterns to those of normal children, i.e. that they have similar phonological processes. Also, they show the persistent use of the common processes of deviant children (*cf.* tables 32, 33). Mentally retarded children, then, appear very like the deviant children with phonological disorders already discussed.

Bangs 1942 is in many ways the most comprehensive of these studies. He studied 53 subjects who were residents of a custodial school. He chose only subjects 'whose speech defects could not be attributed to factors which are known to be of etiological significance in articulatory disorders' (343). They were tested by a naming task, using 65 cards with pictures of common objects. Transcriptions were made at the time of testing.

Bangs analysed the most common substitutions by position and gives figures for the most frequent of them. These data are restated in terms of the processes described in this book and are presented in table 34. They are very similar to the processes used by the deviant children described in section 5.2. This leads Bangs to conclude, 'the sounds most frequently substituted for each sound by the ament also are very similar to those used by the normal child' (356). In section 5.3 it was pointed out that some of the patterns of deviant children were not typically normal

Table 34   The most common substitution processes of 53 mentally retarded children based on Bangs 1942

Processes		Position (% of children using process)		
		Initial	Medial	Final
1 Gliding:	r → w	(60%)	(34%)	(15%)
	l → w	(19%)	(13%)	—
2 Labialization:	θ → f	(49%)	(38%)	(36%)
3 Fronting:	k → t	(25%)	—	(8%)
(Velars)	ŋ → n	—	—	(15%)
4 Stopping:	v → b	(23%)	—	—
	θ → t	—	(32%)	(9%)
	ð → d	—	(43%)	—
	s → t	(13%)	—	—
	ǰ → d	—	(9%)	—
5 Fronting:	š → s	—	(15%)	(15%)
(Palatals)	č → ts	—	(13%)	—
6 Fricatives:	z → s	(11%)	—	—
(Mixed)	θ → s	—	(21%)	(13%)
7 Vocalization	r → Vowel			(11%)
8 Deletion of final consonants				
Stops:	d → ∅			(40%)
	t → ∅			(23%)
	k → ∅			(23%)
	g → ∅			(13%)
	p → ∅			(19%)

Bangs also notes this in his data. 'Many of the minor substitutions made by aments are not in accordance with the usual ones made by children with normal intelligence' (356).

There is one aspect of the data that Bangs feels is especially noteworthy. A large number of the errors are those of omission rather than substitution. Twenty-one per cent of all errors are by omission, and 35 per cent of the final errors are also omissions. 'This fact indicates that omissions are one of the most significant characteristics of the articulating errors found in the feeble-minded' (356). Since data on omissions is not given in the earlier studies, it is not possible to see if this is greater than that done by the deviant children. A glance at the rule system, however, does not show an excessive number of deletion rules. It may be that omissions will prove to be a characteristic of retarded speech. Omission is also found to be a common error pattern in Karlin and Strazzula 1952.

5.43   The hard-of-hearing

Just as the deletion of consonants seems to characterize the speech of the mentally retarded, there appear to be certain characteristics that set the hard-of-hearing apart from both normal and deviant children. Studies of the speech of hard-of-hearing children have been numerous (e.g. Hudgins 1934, Hudgins and Numbers 1942, Carr 1953, Calvert 1962, Fry 1966, John and Howarth 1965, Markides 1970, Levitt and Smith 1972, West and Weber 1973, Oller and Kelly 1974, Oller and Eilers to be published). In these studies, several factors recur indicating that hard-of-hearing speech has a nature of its own.

By far the most extensive of these studies is that of Hudgins and Numbers (1942). In an earlier study, Hudgins (1934) had noted five particular aspects of deaf speech: (*1*) extremely slow, laboured, and excessively breathy speech; (*2*) prolonged production of vowels, resulting in either distortion or the creation of a new syllable; (*3*) a tendency to devoice stops in all positions; (*4*) excessive use of nasality with vowels and consonants; and (*5*) abnormal rhythm across an utterance. The study of Hudgins and Numbers was undertaken to examine more closely the validity of these observations.

Hudgins and Numbers made phonograph recordings of the speech or 192 deaf pupils between 8 and 20 years of age. This resulted in a total of approximately 1200 sentences of 6 to 12 words each. These were examined for the most common errors in both consonants and vowels. They analysed the consonant errors into seven types and the vowel errors into five types. These are shown in table 35 with examples of each process and the percentage of each in terms of total error.

Table 35   Phonological processes used in the speech of deaf children, based on Hudgins and Numbers 1942

Phonological process	Examples		% of total errors (number)
	Consonants		
1 Devoicing of stops $\begin{bmatrix} b \\ d \\ g \\ j \end{bmatrix} \rightarrow \begin{bmatrix} p \\ t \\ t \\ č \end{bmatrix}$	black dog boys food	[pæk] [tak] [pɔys] [fut]	20% (399)
2 Mixed substitutions $r \rightarrow w / \ \# \_$ $l \rightarrow t / V \_ V$ $s \rightarrow y / \ \# \_$ etc.	rode polly Sally	[wout] [pati] [yæli]	7% (149)
3 Cluster reduction (a) Vowel insertion (b) Liquid deletion (c) /s/ deletion	brush fly street	[bərʌš] [fay] [tit]	18% (355)
4 Denasalization $\begin{bmatrix} m \\ n \end{bmatrix} \rightarrow \begin{bmatrix} b \\ d \end{bmatrix}$	summer corner	[sʌmbr̩] [kərtr̩]	12% (225)
5 Vowel insertion, $\emptyset \rightarrow ə / C \_ \$C$ i.e. insert a vowel between two consonants across a syllable ($)	football popcorn on Sunday	[futəbɔl] [papəkɔrn] [anəsʌndey]	6% (121)
6 Final consonant deletion $C \rightarrow \emptyset / \_ \ \#$ (opt.) $C \rightarrow ʔ / \_ \ \#$	race dog Otis	[rey] [da] [owtɪ]	13% (266)
7 Initial consonant deletion $C \rightarrow \emptyset / \ \# \_$	hear go your	[ɪr] [ow] [ɔr]	23% (448)
	Vowels		
1 Substitutions-mixed	beet made team	[bɪt] [mid] [tæm]	55% (444)
2 Simplification of diphthongs (a) Creation of two syllables	boy I	[bawi] [a:i]	9% (72)
(b) Reduce to one vowel	my save	[ma] [sæft]	
3 Creation of two syllables	bread shoes who	[bread] [šuwis] [huwi]	10% (76)
4 Vowel neutralization	will train me	[wʌl] [trʌn] [mʌ]	19% (153)
5 Vowel nasalization			7% (54)

The first striking finding is the large number of errors in the production of vowels. Bangs (1942), for example, finds few vocalic errors in his study, and normal children acquire vowels quite early. Secondly, the devoicing of stops is not like the normal processes of assimilation. Normally stops tend to be voiced before vowels. A third unusual process is the deletion of initial consonants. Normal children usually overcome this quite early. A widespread characteristic of several of the processes is the creation of CV syllables. When two consonants come together, either in a cluster (process 4) or across a syllable boundary (process 5), there is a tendency to insert a [ə] vowel and create a new syllable. This also occurs with vowels where two syllables would be created from one (e.g. *boy* [bawi]). These can be explained as resulting from the earlier noted tendency towards slow, drawn-out speech. This is generally described as inability to produce correct timing in the production of speech (*cf.* John and Howarth 1965).

Since these processes were observed in grouped data, it is probable that deaf children do not individually show all of them. In fact, recent linguistic analyses of younger hard-of-hearing children have shown this. For example, West and Weber (1973) analysed the speech of a girl of 4;4 and found that she had more or less correct use of vowels. At the same time, however, the general tendencies are still evident. Oller and Kelly (1974), for example, noted that a 6-year-old hard-of-hearing girl would avoid final voiced stops by adding a [ə] to the word.

In a study of three young hard-of-hearing children ranging from 5;3 to 6;3 in age, Oller and Eilers (in press) have also confirmed some of Hudgins and Numbers findings. One child, Randy, would break up clusters by the insertion of a [ə], e.g. *block* [bəlɔ́k]. Two of them, Marjie and Melanie, showed a tendency to delete initial consonants. Oller and Eilers compare these deletions to two matched normal children and show that the hard-of-hearing children were deleting them much more frequently. The same two children also showed the addition of syllables, e.g. *baby* [bebeʔe]. This is similar to Hudgins and Numbers findings on the creation of two vowels from one. Markides (1970) has also found cases of this. The same two girls also showed errors in nasalization. Sometimes nasals would replace stops and vice-versa. Hudgins had earlier noted the dimension of nasalization as a particularly striking aspect of hard-of-hearing speech.

While pointing out how hard-of-hearing children differ from other deviant types, it is also important to mention that many of the processes are similar to those of both normal and deviant children. This was emphasized in Oller and Kelly 1974. Also, there is one characteristic that hard-of-hearing children share with deviant children. Oller and Eilers found that the speech of the two young girls was much more unstable than that of two matched normals. This compares favourably with Edwards and Bernhardt's (1973a) findings on deviant children. For example, the girl Marjie showed all the following versions of *pencil*: [bʌ́bɔ, pʌ́bə, pɪ̃tɔ́, étə, péʔtəʔ, pɛd, pɛdə, pédza, pɛ́tɔ́, pʰɛd, pɪa, pɪt, phéʔtʊ́].

5.44   Down's Syndrome

Children with Down's Syndrome are generally considered to have harsh voice qualities (sometimes called 'husky voice'), abnormal intonation, and a pre-dominance of grunts in their speech. Speech production is complicated by the existence of an unusually large tongue. This results in a frequently high level of unintelligibility, and a poor prognosis for ever attaining effective speech (*cf.* Strazzulla 1953).

Recently a detailed linguistic analysis of the speech of two mongoloid boys has appeared by Bodine (1974). Despite the claim that the speech of mongoloid children is by and large gibberish, she found a great deal of systematicity in the speech of the two children, even in their use of grunts. The two subjects were Tommy (5;9) and David (6;2). They were both being raised in their own homes, and neither had the characteristic of 'husky voice'. Spontaneous speech samples were collected in their homes with the use of a tape recorder.

Bodine's analysis differs from several of the analyses of deviant children in that it looks for the phonemic contrasts used in each child's speech (i.e. the organizational level). She also gives examples of the words that the children used. In this way, her analysis is in some ways similar to the one of Ethel in chapter 2.

Tommy's speech was difficult to understand, with an intelligibility rating of only 33 per cent. In those words that were identifiable, there was a great deal of deletion of consonants. The more frequent initial consonants were:

$$
\begin{array}{lll}
\text{b} & \text{d} & \text{g} \\
\text{m} & \text{n} & \\
\text{w} & \text{y} & \\
& & \text{?}
\end{array}
$$

Other consonants were deleted by a process of initial consonant deletion which would also delete initial clusters. The use of nasal consonants and vowels were better aspects of his phonology, although the latter showed a degree of instability. Some substitution patterns for initial consonants were:

Gliding: $r \rightarrow w \, / \, \# \, \_\_$ (opt.)

Glottal replacement: $\left\{ \begin{array}{c} w \\ y \\ h \end{array} \right\} \rightarrow \, ? \, / \, \# \, \_\_$ (optional)

Fronting: $\left\{ \begin{array}{c} k \\ g \end{array} \right\} \rightarrow d \, / \, \# \, \_\_$ (optional)

The use of glottal stops was widespread in Tommy's speech and may be a specific characteristic of mongoloid speech. Some final consonants occurred, although two further processes affected them:

Devoicing $\left[\begin{array}{c} b \\ d \\ g \end{array} \right] \rightarrow \left[\begin{array}{c} p \\ t \\ k \end{array} \right] / \_\_ \, \#$

$\left\{ \begin{array}{c} \text{Fricatives} \\ \text{Affricates} \end{array} \right\} \rightarrow \emptyset \, / \_\_ \, \#$

A particularly perceptive part of the analysis of Tommy's speech is the analysis of his grunts. Bodine found that 25 per cent of his first 270 utterances contained grunts (i.e. glottal stop plus an oral or nasal midfront or midcentral vowel). She divided these into ten categories, the first five being present in the model language. These are summarized in table 36. The samples are usually just one of several alternants used. These are given by Bodine to show the systematicity of the children's grunting.

Table 36   A summary of the communicative grunts used by Tommy, a Down's Syndrome child, based on Bodine 1974

Type of grunt (and number of occurrences)	Example
1 Hesitation grunt, which precedes a following utterance (9)	[ʔə̃ʔ] [ʔababaʰ] *uh, apple pie*
2 A pause filler to mark conversational lull (9)	[ʔɔ̃ʔ] *uh*
3 A grunt in agreement (6)	[ʔoʔ] ([yeəʰ]) *oh yeah*
4 Tag question 'huh' (8)	[hɛ̃h] *huh?*
5 Concentration sounds (17)	[ʔəʔə]
6 Preface to demonstration (6) (meaning 'I'll show you')	[ʔə<]
7 Pointing (2)	[ʔɔ̃ʔɔ̃]
8 Objecting (3)	[ʔiʔiʔiʔi]
9 Commanding (6)	[(də)ʔəˇ(dəʔ)ʔɛ·]
10 Giving in after first disagreeing (2)	[ʔɛʔɛʰ]

David's speech was much more developed than Tommy's (intelligibility set at 75 per cent). Consequently he sounded much more like a normal child. His speech showed a number of common phonological processes. Initial consonants were generally well pronounced, with a few substitutions (i.e. [č] to [d] or [z], [v] → ∅, [ð] → [d], [š] → [s]). Final voiced stops and voiced fricatives were deleted. This appears to be a persistent process in that initial consonants and even consonant clusters were reasonably well-developed. Vocalization occurred where [r] → [i].

Bodine presents a detailed analysis of David's production of consonant clusters in initial medial, and final positions. A summary of his treatment of initial clusters follows to show how common processes are being used.

Adult	David	Processes
/tr–/	f	Assimilation of obstruent in cluster
/fr–/	fw	Gliding
/s/ + Stop	correct	
/s/ + Continuant	s	Liquid deletion
C + /$\left\{{l \atop r}\right\}$/	C	Liquid deletion

David, who does not rely on grunts, shows many of the normal phonological processes, although in what may be a deviant system through the persistence of individual processes.

5.45   Cleft palate

Each of the two preceding disorders shows a distinctive articulation feature resulting from the organic damage. The hard-of-hearing show drawn-out arhymthmic speech with distorted voice quality; the Down's Syndrome child produces in its more severe forms a larger number of grunts. Cleft palate children also show a particular effect on their speech resulting from organic damage. This effect is the nasalization of their speech sounds. Whereas the other disorders are directly reflected in delayed speech, the picture is not so clear in children with cleft palates. One may ask whether the occurrence of a cleft not only affects the child's speech, but also results in delayed speech.

Morley (1966) has suggested that cleft palate children go through a period of defective speech between 3 and 6, but that these errors are spontaneously corrected. Some studies, however, have suggested otherwise. Both Bzoch (1965) and Philips and Harrison (1969) have found that cleft palate children at the ages of 5 and 6 do not do as well as a group as three-year-old normal children. The occurrence of a cleft palate, then, can generally be considered as causing a delay in articulation development.

The next question is whether the delay is normal, or whether these children show deviance in the sense of section 5.34. Several studies have examined the speech patterns of cleft palate children, e.g. Byrne *et al.* 1961, Spriesterbach *et al.* 1956, Bzoch 1965, Moll 1968, and Philips and Harrison 1969, although no linguistic analyses of individual children have appeared. Spriesterbach *et al.* (1956) studied the speech of 25 cleft lip and/or palate children between 3;7 and 8;3 (mean IQ 115). The subjects were given the Templin–Darley Test. The easiest sounds for the children were [m], [n], [ŋ], [h], [y]. The most difficult sounds were the fricatives and affricates (with the exception of [v] and [f]). This is consistent with our results with deviant children in which fricatives and affricates were among the most difficult sounds to produce. The cleft palate children had difficulty with clusters, and showed a general inconsistency in their misarticulations. These children, then, appear to be very similar to other deviant children. Similar error patterns were also found by Byrne *et al.* (1961).

Philips and Harrison (1969) pursued this further in a study matching the cleft palate children with normal controls. They matched 74 cleft palate children (all with clefts of the soft palate) to normal children of the same ages. There were four groups: 2;0–2;11 (N = 10); 3;0–3;11 (27); 4;0–4;11 (16); 5;0–5;11 (21). All subjects received an articulation test with 100 items. There were sufficient similarities in the error patterns for the authors to conclude: 'the articulation error patterns of the cleft palate subjects suggest a generalized delay in development' (251). The errors of the cleft palate children, however, differed in two ways. First, they showed more errors in medial consonants than initial ones, while the normal had equal errors in both. Secondly, 'substitution errors did not decrease appreciably with chronological age for cleft palate children as they did for the normal children' (250). In discussing the latter, they say, 'the cleft palate subjects either are correcting only errors of omission or ... these are being commuted to substitutions and indistinct productions' (252). This suggests the persistence of processes that characterizes deviant speech.

5.5   Summary

It is important to establish how the phonology of children with a disorder differs from that of normal children. This can be done by the examination of several analyses of the speech of deviant children and a comparison with what is known about normal development. Children who have language disorders can be placed into two broad classifications: those who have a problem because of a known organic cause, e.g. deafness, cleft palate etc., and those who appear normal in terms of intellectual, aural, and social development, but who nonetheless have a language problem. For want of a better term, the latter are often called 'deviant', in that their language deviates from the normal process. The question of comparison with normal development needs to be considered separately for each of these two groups.

Phonological analyses of deviant children have been made by Hinckley (1915) and Haas (1963), and more recently by Compton (1970, 1975), Pollock and Rees (1972), Oller *et al.* (1972), Oller (1973), Edwards and Bernhardt (1973a), and Lorentz (1972, 1974). Although these studies vary greatly in their approach and the data presented, there is sufficient information in them to answer some of the fundamental questions.

First, it is clear from these studies that the phonologies of these children are systematic. They show the use of sounds to contrast the meanings of words, and they use a variety of phonological processes to simplify the production of words. Their phonologies are not, however, the same as those of younger normal children. For one thing, they sometimes use processes that are not commonly or widely used by normal children. For example, a process that a normal child may use for a short time in a few words may be used by a deviant child for a long time in a large number of words. Particularly, the more severely affected children may use simplifying processes that the normal child often need not resort to, e.g. the stopping of liquids. Also, processes do not appear to drop out in the same order as they do for normal children. Certain processes tend to *persist*, eventually cooccurring with those more characteristic of older children's speech. Children differ as to which processes persist, although certain ones occur very frequently. Those used to simplify the production of fricatives and affricates appear to be among the most persistent.

Children with organic causes of speech disorder also show similar systems to deviant children, although they may show individual peculiarities. This is particularly true of the hard-of-hearing, who show unusually striking difficulties with vowels and syllables. They tend to produce CV syllables by several different means. Down's Syndrome is often characterized by grunts, but these grunts can be shown to be systematic.

6

Issues in remediation

6.1 Explicitly principled therapy

In the first chapter it was emphasized that the primary contribution of linguistics lies in the establishment of an explicitly principled therapy. Through an accurate diagnosis of the child's phonological system, we will know where the child's problem lies. Haas (1963) summed up this point nicely:

> The contribution of linguistics is chiefly diagnostic. A linguistic diagnosis will contribute towards working out a rational sequence of therapeutic steps: i.e. a sequence which is adapted to the requirements of the individual case and which embodies a scale of priorities according to the relative seriousness of the defects to be treated. (246)

Therapy will be based on the individual child's needs, according to the linguistic analysis of his speech and what is known about the process of acquisition.

Chapters 2 to 5 have provided information helpful in constructing an explicit therapy. It has been shown that the child does not acquire sounds in isolation, but deals with phonological processes that affect entire classes of sound. Training, therefore cannot deal with isolated sounds but rather with general processes. Much of the earlier presentation has dealt with the determining of phonological processes in children's speech, and it is these which are the targets of therapy. Next, there is the question of how to attack individual processes. For example, many processes affect only one articulatory feature of sounds. For example, stopping in some cases will change fricative to [–continuant], i.e. stops. Is it possible then, to teach anyone of the sounds affected by process, e.g. [s] → [t], with the expectation that once one is eliminated the rest of the sounds will be correct? Compton (1970), for example, has suggested that this is the case. This suggestion, which can be called the Generalization Hypothesis, will be discussed in some detail in 6.23.

Even when processes and a procedure for their elimination are determined, there are still other facts that can make the therapy more explicit. The point has been made that phonology is a system of contrasts. If a child's own system lacks certain contrasts, they will need to be targets of therapy. Here aspects to be concentrated upon are the instability of the child's production and the elimination of homonyms. These changes will lead to the effective use of contrasts. This is related to the issue of what to teach first. There are various ways to decide this, including selecting those processes that result in the most homonyms, those that render speech most unintelligible etc. The factors involved in this decision are the focus of 6.4.

Lastly, there are two further facts that demand attention. First, normal acquisition is gradual. That is, the child acquires a sound in time by stages. Should we expect the deviant child to be different? If not, we need to revise our definition of correctness and assume success if the child proceeds to the next stage, even if the production is still not correct by adult standards. Secondly, what is the role of perception in speech training? Does training in discrimination of sounds come before production?

These are some of the facts that can lead to an explicitly principled therapy. It is therapy based on the child's system and expectations of how the system will function and develop. The goals at each step will be explicit, and consequently the success or failure at each step may be evaluated. Attempts at therapy in turn will establish which steps are ultimately successful and which are not.

6.2 The elimination of phonological processes

6.21 The inadequacy of substitution analyses

Much of the discussion of the many phonological processes in child phonology has been directed at demonstrating the inadequacy of substitution analysis. For example, the Templin–Darley Test was criticized because it assumes that children learn language on a sound-by-sound basis. Thus, therapy, on the same assumption, can be considered as simply teaching the substitution of a correct sound for an incorrect one. All analyses of children's acquisition have shown this to be wrong. Children show very general processes that affect whole classes of sound.

This can be exemplified by looking at Jim's rule of assimilation (*cf.* table 26), which is repeated below:

$$\begin{bmatrix} t \\ d \end{bmatrix} \rightarrow \begin{bmatrix} k \\ g \end{bmatrix} / - V \begin{Bmatrix} k \\ g \end{Bmatrix}$$

Hypothetical examples (since Compton did not give any) would be *dog* [gɔg] and *tick* [kɪk]. A substitution approach would be to deal with [t] and [d] separately as if they were not related. The fact that both change in this way shows that they only change in this one specific place, i.e. when followed by a velar stop. What needs to be eliminated here is not an idiosyncratic tendency to replace [t] and [d] randomly with [k] and [g] respectively, but rather a very systematic and general process of assimilation.

Another example would be the case of a child who says [gɪk] for *tick*. The substitution analysis approach would be to teach the child to say [t] instead of [g]. In reality, however, two processes are involved: velar assimilation and voicing of a consonant before a vowel. If the former is corrected, [dɪk] will be produced; if the latter [kɪk]. By focusing on the individual processes, training will concentrate on several sounds within a class, rather than a sound by sound basis. Elimination of a single process will have a much wider effect on the child's system than the teaching of an individual sound affected by several processes. The diagnosis of the child's phonology into a set of phonological processes provides the general patterns of the child's speech which need to be eliminated.

The specification of phonological processes also makes it possible to determine sounds which are the result of substitution versus sounds which result from processes. For example, a deviant child, Aaron, at 3;11, gave the following pronunciations of words beginning with word initial [d]:

deer	[dir]		*door*	[dow]
desk	[sʌk]		*dress*	[sæs]
doctor	[gago]		*drum*	[lam]
dog	[kak]		*duck*	[gʌk]
	[dɔk]			
	[gak]			

In a substitution analysis, one would simply give the various substitutions, i.e. /d-/ = [d] 3, [g] 3, [k] 3, [s] 2, and [l] 1. The result would be that /d/ is substituted for 75 per cent of the time. A closer analysis in terms of processes, however, shows that Aaron can pronounce [d]. It does not occur in all cases, however, because of the following:

Velar assimilation: *doctor, dog, duck*
s salience: *dress, desk*
Deletion of unmarked member of cluster: *drum* ([r] → [l] here)

These processes affect segments other than just /d/ and are general aspects of his system. The partial use of [d], as a result, is not due to substitutions but to processes.

6.22 The use of distinctive features

Phonological processes throughout this book have been described by showing the segments that were affected. Many of the analyses from which they were taken, however, stated them in terms of their distinctive features. Since this method of representing processes has been claimed as important in planning therapy, it is necessary to take a closer look at it.

Individual sounds can be described in terms of their articulatory features. Also, since any feature is or is not part of a sound it can be considered binary, i.e. plus ' + ' or minus '—'. For example, the segment [t] can be considered. (For the sake of clarity, I will use features which are not necessarily those currently employed in linguistic theory):

$$[t] = \begin{bmatrix} + \text{ consonant} \\ - \text{ vowel} \\ + \text{ stop} \\ + \text{ alveolar} \end{bmatrix}$$

Features are used so that generality can be captured. Sounds fall into what are called *natural classes*, such as consonants, vowels etc. A natural class is a class of sounds that can be described by fewer features than any of its members. For example, consonants can be described as [+ consonant] [—vowel], while more features would be needed to specify any particular consonant. A rule stated in features will show how general it is. The fewer features in the rule, the wider application, i.e. the more segments it affects.

Also, by use of features it is possible to show which feature is changing in a phonological process. For example, below is the rule of prevocalic voicing stated in segments and features:

$$\begin{bmatrix} P \\ t \\ k \end{bmatrix} \rightarrow \begin{bmatrix} b \\ d \\ g \end{bmatrix} / \# \_ V \qquad \begin{bmatrix} + \text{ consonant} \\ + \text{ stop} \\ - \text{ voice} \end{bmatrix} \rightarrow [+ \text{ voice}] / \# \_ \begin{bmatrix} + \text{ vowel} \\ + \text{ voice} \end{bmatrix}$$

The feature rule explicitly shows that only the features [± voice] change, and also that it is assimilation because the following segment is [+ voice]. The use of features allows for the explicit statement of the changes in phonological rules whereas it is only implicitly shown in rules given in segments.

6.221 Features as a descriptive device

The use of features has characterized much of the work of linguists in recent years in the area of phonology. This is because features are very effective means of describing a phonological pattern. Since linguists are concerned with determining how speakers capture generalization, they are very concerned with making description more explicit.

Take, for example, the first two rules for Tom as given in table 25. The linguist would not be content with them in segments. They would be rewritten:

(*i*) $\begin{Bmatrix} č \\ š \end{Bmatrix} \rightarrow s$ $\quad \begin{bmatrix} + \text{ consonant} \\ + \text{ strident} \\ + \text{ alveopalatal} \\ - \text{ voice} \end{bmatrix} \rightarrow \begin{bmatrix} + \text{ alveolar} \\ - \text{ alveopalatal} \end{bmatrix}$

(*ii*) $\begin{array}{l} f \rightarrow t \\ s \rightarrow t \\ j \rightarrow d \end{array}$ $\quad \begin{bmatrix} + \text{ consonant} \\ + \text{ strident} \\ - \text{ velar} \\ \langle + \text{ alveopalatal} \rangle \\ \langle + \text{ voice} \rangle \end{bmatrix} \rightarrow \begin{bmatrix} + \text{ alveolar} \\ - \text{labiodental} \\ + \text{ stop} \\ \langle + \text{voice} \rangle \end{bmatrix}$

The angle brackets in rule (*ii*) are a formal device which indicate that when the features inside them on the left occur, the change on the right must also occur. Also, in an attempt to capture even greater generality, the linguist would use features different from the straightforward ones I have given. There can be no question therefore that features are a useful descriptive device.

Learning to use features, however, requires a certain amount of study. (A fine introduction to the subject can be found in Schane 1973.) Also, showing a rule in features is an abstraction and consequently takes one away from the actual segments. When a rule is presented in features, it takes time to reconstruct the segments to which it actually refers. Because of this, a better use of features is to show them side by side with the rule in segments so that one can see both the segments and the explicit generalization through features. Because of the additional training necessary, the question can be raised whether or not a clinician needs to know how to use features in order to describe a child's language. That is, while the needs of the linguist require the use of features, do the needs of the clinician?

This is an important question that is not always explicitly discussed in articles. Oller (1973) suggests the use of features in describing abnormal phonologies because they are a more effective *descriptive device*. However, it is not clear that this is a sufficient reason for their use by clinicians. For example, observe the rule of prevocalic voicing shown above in segments and features. Anyone with a basic knowledge of phonetics will be able to understand the generality of the process as stated in segments. While features make the process more explicit, they do not necessarily add new information. In the second rule from Tom just given, the same is also true. The feature rule describes the process more explicitly, but it does not necessarily add new information. Also, if the three parts of this rule differed in their optionality, the use of features would create difficulties in trying to show this. For this reason, while knowledge of features would be helpful to a clinician for descriptive purposes, it is not essential.

There is, however, another reason put forward for the use of features. This is that the description of a rule in features makes predictions about how that process can be changed through therapy (*cf.* Compton 1970). It is this suggestion that has important implications and has been the focus of several research studies of late.

6.222   Features as a predictive device

There are two ways that features may be taken as a predictive device. The first, and the strongest, would be that children acquire language by acquiring features, not segments, and that a rule in features *predicts* future changes. For example, Applegate (1961) describes the use of initial fricatives and affricates by three boys, ages 4, 5;6 and 8;6 respectively. The children's substitutions were:

Adult	Child		Adult	Child
/f-/	[p]		/s-/	[t]
/v-/	[b]		/z-/	[t]
/θ-/	[t]		/š-/	[t]
/ð-/	[d]		/č-/	[t]
			/ǰ-/	[dt]

These can be shown by two processes in segments:

Fronting of palatals:
$$\begin{bmatrix} \text{š} \\ \text{č} \\ \text{ǰ} \end{bmatrix} \rightarrow \begin{bmatrix} \text{s} \\ \text{ts} \\ \text{dz} \end{bmatrix} / \# \underline{\quad}$$

Stopping:
$$\begin{bmatrix} f \\ \left\{\begin{matrix} \theta \\ s \\ ts \end{matrix}\right\} \end{bmatrix} \rightarrow \begin{bmatrix} p \\ t \end{bmatrix} \bigg/ \# \underline{} \qquad \begin{bmatrix} v \\ \left\{\begin{matrix} \eth \\ z \\ dz \end{matrix}\right\} \end{bmatrix} \rightarrow \begin{bmatrix} b \\ d \end{bmatrix} \bigg/ \# \underline{}$$

In segments, the rules are direct but cumbersome, in that it requires several symbols. In features, however, both can be collapsed into one:

$$\begin{bmatrix} + \text{ consonant} \\ + \text{ fricative} \\ \langle + \text{ alveopalatal}\rangle a \\ \langle + \text{ dental}\rangle a \\ \langle + \text{ labiodental}\rangle b \end{bmatrix} \rightarrow \begin{bmatrix} - \text{ fricative} \\ \langle + \text{ alveolar}\rangle a \\ \langle + \text{ labial}\rangle b \end{bmatrix} \bigg/ \# \underline{}$$

where [— fricative] is taken to mean [+ stop]. The rule reduce these to one manner, i.e. stops, and two places, labial and alveolar. If children acquire features, not segments, the prediction would be that when [+ fricative] is acquired by the child, it would influence all the segments. The child would then have the following system:

Adult	Child	Adult	Child
/f/	[ø]	/z/	[s]
/v/	[β]	/š/	[s]
/θ/	[s]	/č/	[s]
/ð/	[z]	/ǰ/	[z]
/s/	[s]		

Children do not, however, acquire fricatives in this fashion. Each segment appears to have its own development, although there are some acquisitions that seem to affect more than one segment. For example, table 37 shows Smith's son's initial fricatives and affricates at five different ages. There is some spread of features here. For example, at 2;11 to 3;0 frication is being acquired for the palatal, alveolar and dental sounds. At each step, however, there are individual variations. In the first period, /f/ and /v/ are continuants but the others are not. In the second one, [f] appears, but not other fricatives. Also, /z/ shows [r]. Through the entire five ages /ð/ is stopped and does not fall in line. Evidence like this suggests

Table 37   A's fricatives and affricates at five ages

Adult	2;2–2;5	2;10	2;11–3;0	3;1	3;9–3;11
/f/	w	f	f	f	f
/v-/	v, w	v, w	v, w	v, w	v, w
/θ-/	d	t	t, ts, s	s	s
/ð-/	d	d	d	d	d
/s-/	d	t	t, ts, s	s	s
/z-/	d	r	r	z	z
/š-/	d	t	t, ts, s	s	š
/č-/	d	t	ts	s	č
/ǰ-/	d	d	d, dz	d, dz	dz

that children do not acquire features across the board, but rather individually within segments. (This, in fact, is essentially the position of Crocker (1969), as I understand it.)

Since fricatives are complicated in terms of features, and the feature [+ fricative] does not adequately capture them (e.g. [s], [z] are [+ spirant] but [θ], [ð] are [− spirant]), one could argue that a better feature analysis might reflect the acquisition of features. Another and perhaps more clear-cut example would be the devoicing of final consonants. Suppose a child has the following rule:

$$
\begin{bmatrix} b \\ d \\ g \end{bmatrix} \rightarrow \begin{bmatrix} p \\ t \\ k \end{bmatrix} / \underline{\quad} \# \qquad \begin{bmatrix} + \text{ consonant} \\ + \text{ stop} \\ + \text{ voice} \end{bmatrix} \rightarrow [- \text{ voice}] / \underline{\quad} \#
$$

For this rule to be predictive, it would suggest that final voicing would occur for all stops at the same time. Evidence contrary to this would indicate that it may vary from segment to segment. Data on more limited cases like this are not as clear on this issue. It may be that for certain limited processes a feature description may predict the future change.

Overall, however, most analyses of children's speech show that segments are handled separately. For example, in Tom's second rule (table 25), the process of stopping is optional for [s], but obligatory for [f], and [ʃ], even though all three undergo the process. This conclusion was summed up nicely by Moskowitz (1970) in describing her analysis of the phonology of a child named Mackie:

> . . . *the learning of distinctive features per se is not a primary goal of Mackie's linguistic practice at this time.* Once learned, then, a feature does not necessarily spread rapidly throughout the system to all relevant segments. (431)

The second related and weaker form of prediction is that a child's rule in features can be used to teach generalization in a clinical setting. For example, if a child has the above rule devoicing final voiced stops, clinically he would only need to be taught one of these. Once it is taught, it presumably will generalize to other segments. This use of features has been recently advocated by Compton (1970).

6.23   The generalization hypothesis

Compton (1970) explicitly points out that he advocates the use of features for clinical as well as descriptive purposes. 'Over and above the gains in descriptive adequacy resulting from the analyses presented here are the clinical implications which follow from the generalizations that have been made' (331). Without justifying this principle with observations on language acquisition, he proceeds to cite the generalization principle, referring to rule C (*cf.* 5.22 in this book): 'the "correction" of this misarticulation for any one sound within the class will automatically result in a correction of the remaining class members. Consequently, there would be little need to work with more than one of the sounds within the class' (331).

In the last part of the article, Compton outlines how therapy would proceed on the basis of this assumption. He focuses specifically on Jim's inability to produce word final nasals (*cf.* table 26). The clinician working with Jim only trained for the production of final /–m/. No other nasals were taught. After about two weeks the clinician also attempted to eliminate Jim's nasalization of vowels (*cf.* rule iv, table 26). This again was only attempted before the nasal /–m/. If children do acquire features, then the correction of both of these processes with /–m/ should also generalize to other nasals. After five weeks Jim was retested on the same articulation test. Of the 17 words with final nasals (6 for /n/ and /ŋ/, 5 for /m/), there was not a single one showing either of these processes. Compton takes this as evidence of the predictive value of features in planning therapy.

Since Jim was already producing some final nasals, and he was only tested on this process, this evidence must be interpreted cautiously. Fortunately, Compton (1975) has provided more extensive data on this approach with a child called Frank, allowing a closer evaluation of the generalization hypothesis.

The main phonological processes in Frank's system have already been provided in table 27. Compton reports on a therapy programme that was undertaken with Frank and evaluated at six different periods. The programme did not attack all processes at once, but selected particular ones for each session. As processes were eliminated, new ones were taken on. With those processes that affected more than one segment, the generalization hypothesis was tested by training in one of the sounds only. The periodic evaluations made it possible to see whether generalization was taking place to the other segments of the process.

There were two clearcut cases where generalization appeared to work. In the first period of therapy, the /s/ loss part of cluster reduction was trained (*cf.* table 27, Compton's rule 11) by only working on /sp–/ clusters:

Original sample	*Evaluation 1*	*Evaluation 2*
s → ∅ / __ C (oblig.)	s → ∅ / __ C (opt. 20%)[1]	process eliminated

Although training was only done on /sp/ clusters, the use of /s/ appeared before other consonants. The other case involved Frank's affrication rule (Compton's rule 3).

Original sample	*Evaluation 2*
$\begin{bmatrix} t \\ d \end{bmatrix} \rightarrow \begin{bmatrix} č \\ ǰ \end{bmatrix}$ / __ rV	process eliminated

Therapy on this process was undertaken in the second therapy period and was eliminated by the second evaluation.

There were two other cases that suggested generalization although other complicating factors were involved. One of these was the devoicing of final stops process. In the first period, Frank was trained only on final [b]. In the second and third periods, however, training was shifted to [g]. Consequently, two of the three segments affected were trained, not just one.

---

[1] '(opt. 20%)' indicates that process is now optional, occurring in 20% of the possible instances where it could apply.

Original sample	Evaluation 1	Evaluation 2	Evaluation 3
$\begin{bmatrix} b \\ d \\ g \end{bmatrix} \rightarrow \begin{bmatrix} p \\ t \\ k \end{bmatrix} /\_\# \ (\text{opt.})$	$\begin{bmatrix} b \\ d \\ g \end{bmatrix} \rightarrow \begin{bmatrix} bp \\ dt \\ gk \end{bmatrix} /\_\# \ (\text{opt.})$	$\begin{bmatrix} b \\ d \\ g \end{bmatrix} \rightarrow \begin{bmatrix} bp \\ dt \\ gk \end{bmatrix} /\_\# \ (\text{opt.})$	Process Eliminated
90% occurrence	90% occurrence	50% occurrence	

The second case deals with the teaching of cluster reduction of liquids. /r/ was taught in /tr-/ in the second period, and in /br-/ in the third. The use generalized to all /r/ clusters in the third evaluation. Liquid clusters with /l/ were trained in the third period with only /bl/ and were eliminated by the third evaluation. There were, however, C/l/ clusters occurring in the second evaluation, these in turn the result of individual work on /l/ as a single segment. These cases are not as clear since training involved more than one context of the processes.

Despite the above supportive evidence, there are also three cases where the prediction of generalization did not work. Each of these involved training on pairs of fricatives or affricates. In period 4 the clinician attempted to eliminate Frank's initial stopping of the dental fricatives. This was done by training only /ð/. This resulted, however, only in changes of /ð/ and not /θ/.

Original	Evaluation 4	Evaluation 5
$\begin{bmatrix} \theta \\ \delta \end{bmatrix} \rightarrow \begin{bmatrix} t \\ d \end{bmatrix} /\#\_$ (oblig.)	$\begin{bmatrix} \theta \\ \delta \end{bmatrix} \rightarrow \begin{bmatrix} t \\ d \end{bmatrix} /\#\_ \begin{array}{l}(\text{opt. }75\%) \\ (\text{opt. }40\%)\end{array}$	$\begin{bmatrix} \theta \\ \delta \end{bmatrix} \rightarrow \begin{bmatrix} t \\ d \end{bmatrix} /\#\_ \begin{array}{l}(\text{opt. }75\%) \\ (\text{opt. }10\%)\end{array}$

The other two cases affected final segments. In period 3, the elimination of the process that reduced final affricates to fricatives was attempted by training /ǰ/. This, however, affected primarily this segment.

Original	Evaluation 3	Evaluation 4
$\begin{bmatrix} \check{c} \\ \check{j} \end{bmatrix} \rightarrow$ fricatives (oblig.)	$\begin{bmatrix} \check{c} \\ \check{j} \end{bmatrix} \rightarrow$ fricatives $\begin{array}{l}(70\%) \\ (10\%)\end{array}$ (opt.)	$\check{c} \rightarrow \check{s}$ (opt. 20%) Process eliminated for /ǰ-/

Finally, at period 4, an attempt was made to train word final dental fricatives by focusing on /θ/. As a result, /ð/ was not affected.

Evaluation 3	Evaluation 4	Evaluation 5
$\begin{bmatrix} \theta \\ \delta \end{bmatrix} \rightarrow \begin{bmatrix} s \\ v \end{bmatrix} /\_\# \begin{array}{l}(\text{opt. }60\%) \\ (\text{oblig.})\end{array}$	$\begin{bmatrix} \theta \\ \delta \end{bmatrix} \rightarrow \begin{bmatrix} f \\ v \end{bmatrix} /\_\# \begin{array}{l}(\text{opt. }60\%) \\ (\text{opt. }75\%)\end{array}$	$\begin{bmatrix} \theta \\ \delta \end{bmatrix} \rightarrow \begin{bmatrix} f \\ v \end{bmatrix} /\_\# \begin{array}{l}(\text{opt. }20\%) \\ (\text{opt. }75\%)\end{array}$

These cast serious doubt on the effectiveness of teaching for generalization.

There is still another piece of evidence which casts doubts on the validity of the generalization approach: several of Frank's processes improved spontaneously without any therapy at all. It is possible that the changes that took place with generalization may have occurred spontaneously. Some of the processes that changed without therapy are:

Assimilation: $\begin{bmatrix} t \\ d \end{bmatrix} \rightarrow \begin{bmatrix} k \\ g \end{bmatrix} / \# \underline{\quad} V \begin{Bmatrix} k \\ g \end{Bmatrix}$ opt.

10%	Disappeared at Evaluation 1
s → š / # __ (opt. 20%)	Disappeared at Evaluation 2
š → s / # __ (opt. 50%)	Disappeared at Evaluation 2
w → ∅ / f __ (oblig.)	Disappeared at Evaluation 3
š → s / __ # (opt. 90%)	Disappeared at Evaluation 3

Although the first two had low percentages of occurrence, the latter did not. These suggest that changes were occurring throughout the child's system and it is not always clear which were the result of therapy. Overall, the data does not provide convincing evidence that the generalization hypothesis is correct.

A study which provides more supportive evidence for this hypothesis is that by McReynolds and Bennett 1972, itself an extension of McReynolds and Huston 1971. McReynolds and Bennett investigated 'the generality of features' (464). They wanted to determine whether training one segment of a process would result in generalization to another segment of the process. They also wanted to see if generalization would occur in initial and final word positions. They did this by first teaching the child the consonant selected in the initial position of a nonsense syllable. When this was achieved, training switched to the final position of the nonsense syllable. (See McReynolds and Bennett 1972, 464–5, for the details of the training procedure.) At various points testing for generalization was done by giving the child selected parts of the McDonald Test.

The authors present data from three children who were taught features in this fashion. Subject 1 did not produce strident sounds, i.e. [f], [s], [z], [č], [v]. He was taught this feature through the segment [f]. When tested to see if his training resulted in generalization to other strident sounds, he showed the following results in terms of percentage correctly produced:

Subject 1	% before training	% after training
f	0	98
v	0	47
s	0	100
z	0	60
č	0	94
θ	0	0

The [θ] shows that only strident sounds were affected. A second subject showed errors on the feature of voicing in stops. To train this, the sound [b] was selected, and the following results obtained:

Subject 2	% before training	% after training
b	7	85
d	0	87
g	0	87

Like subject 1, subject 2 showed generalization to other segments. A last subject is presented who had difficulty with the feature continuancy with fricatives. Presumably the subject showed a process of stopping. This was trained by using the segment /š/.

Subject 3	% before training	% after training
š	0	92
s	0	92
z	0	36
f	0	64
v	0	60

The generalization was less dramatic here, especially for /z/, and yet distinct changes did take place.

Compton (1975) found that there was little evidence from Frank's speech suggesting that the use of a sound would generalize from initial to final position. McReynolds and Bennett, however, tested for generalization of this kind. The percentages of correct production given above reflect the use in both positions combined. Regarding differences between initial and final position, they state: 'Some children generalized to both positions equally. Some, however, generalized almost completely to one position, but negligibly to the others' (470).

Results like this suggest that generalization may take place under carefully controlled conditions. While one would like to see if the correct productions extended to spontaneous speech, these results suggest that the generalization hypothesis is worthy of continued research.

6.24   Summary

It is clear from several recent studies that phonological processes need to be the target of therapy, rather than unrelated sounds. In training out processes there are two possible ways in which a clinician may proceed. One is to teach all the segments of the process at the same time. The other is to teach only one of the segments, based on the assumption that features are acquired, not segments. The acquisition of a new feature will spread to other segments affected by the process. This assumption has yet to be proven empirically. Data from normal acquisition suggests that children do not acquire features across the board, but segments. Even cases where features appear to be acquired often show the segments with different percentages of occurrence. Results from studies specifically attempting to teach features have been mixed. Data from Compton 1970, 1975 have not been convincing. Stronger support comes from controlled study by McReynolds and Bennett (1972).

Given the uncertainty of the generalization hypothesis, it appears to be best to take a conservative position on it at the present time. In this case then, it is probably safer to attack a process by training on all the affected segments, until more is known about the nature and limitations of generalization of features. This, in fact, is what has been suggested by Edwards and Bernhardt (1973a). As research continues on generalization, it is to be hoped that it will also become incorporated into therapy, since it suggests a method of instituting broad changes in a child's system with a relative minimum of training.

6.3 The establishment of contrasts

The acquisition of phonology is concerned with the acquisition of the ability to use sounds contrastively. In attacking phonological processes, one is eliminating the child's tendency to simplify speech. At the same time, it is important to assist the child to use more and more sounds contrastively, i.e. to mark one word as different from another. The focus should not be just on the elimination of one systematic aspect of linguistic behaviour, but also on the establishment of new behaviour. As the child acquires new ways to contrast speech sounds, he will be able to attain higher degrees of intelligibility.

There are three basic ways that the deviant child's speech is deficient in the use of contrast. One is the unstable use of speech. As noted by Oller and Eilers (1975) and Edwards and Bernhardt (1973a), some deviant children can show a great deal of phonetic alternation in their words. This makes it very difficult for the adults in their lives to determine the manner in which they reduce speech. As a result, it creates a very unintelligible language system. Another is the use of a large number of homonyms. If the child uses one utterance as a form to refer to many different adult words, interpretation becomes a matter of guesswork. Lastly, the child's system may have a small inventory of contrastive elements. These would need to be increased before more effective speech can occur. There are three crucial aspects of a child's phonology that should be a central part of remedial therapy.

6.31 The elimination of instability

If a deviant child in therapy shows a great deal of phonetic variation, this in itself needs to be one of the goals of therapy. One obvious way to reduce variation is to have the child simply pronounce the words of his vocabulary correctly. Although this may sometimes be attempted, in reality it is a very unrealistic goal as a first step. There is, however, a much more direct and feasible alternative. This is first to *stabilize the child's own contrastive form of a word.*

Earlier, the following pronunciations were noted by Oller and Eilers (1975) for a young hard-of-hearing girl's production of *pencil*:

(1) [bʌbɔ]	(5) [pɛ́ʔtəʔ]	(9) [pɛ́tə]	(13) [pʰɛ́ʔtʊ́]
(2) [pʌ́bə]	(6) [pɛd]	(10) [pʰad]	
(3) [pĭtə]	(7) [pɛdə]	(11) [pɪa]	
(4) [ɛ́tə]	(8) [pɛdza]	(12) [pɪt]	

These show several processes in operation: labial assimilations (1, 2), consonant deletions (4, 11), syllable deletions (6, 10, 12), and vowel variations (1, 2, 3, 10, 12). Across all these, the child's target or 'underlying form' (in the sense of her organization system) is /pɛtə/. This then would show stopping, vocalization, de-aspiration, and nasal cluster deletion:

[pʰɛnsḷ]	*Adult form*
pʰentḷ	Stopping
pʰentə	Vocalization
pʰɛtə	Nasal cluster reduction
pɛtə	Loss of aspiration
[pɛtə]	*Child's form*

While these processes will be targets of therapy, their elimination will be troublesome as long as other minor processes interrupt them.

The goal with this form would be to stabilize her use of the word as [pɛtə]. This could be done by either directly eliciting it or by accepting it when pronounced but rejecting other alternatives. This in turn becomes an effective way of eliminating the minor processes mentioned above. Since processes like these are usually sporadic and unpredictable, it is hard to attack them directly. Once the stable use of /pɛtə/ occurs, then the child has these segments available for contrast. For example, this word may be used in contrast to [bɛtə] for *better* or other possible forms (e.g. *puzzle* [pʌtə]). Also, once stabilized, the major processes shown in the above derivation from the adult to the child form are isolated and exposed for direct therapy.

6.32   The elimination of homonyms

Ingram (1975c) found that normal children use fewer homonyms than expected: in other words, they are reasonably effective in using sounds to keep words separate from each other. Section 5.33 discussed this and mentioned that the use of homonyms may be more widespread in deviant speech. The following example was given from Aaron, a deviant child who was 3;11 at the time of sampling.

$$\frac{butter, \; ladder, \; letter, \; spider}{water, \; whistle} = [dado]$$

Because [dado] could mean so many different things, its use could easily lead to misunderstanding.

In cases like these, the form with so many meanings should be a major target of therapy. This could be done by selecting those processes for therapy that are creating the greatest use of homonymy. In Aaron's example, the following distinctions could be established by eliminating processes one by one:

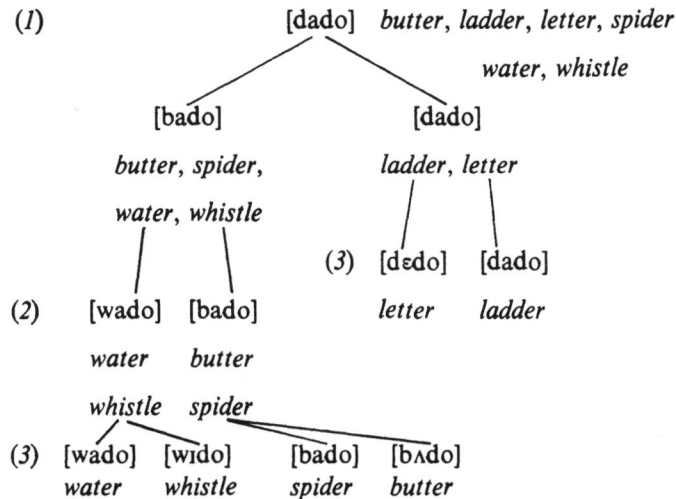

(1)   [dado]   *butter, ladder, letter, spider*

water, whistle

[bado]   [dado]

butter, spider,   *ladder, letter*

water, whistle

                 (3)   [dɛdo]   [dado]

(2)   [wado]   [bado]   *letter*   *ladder*

water   *butter*

whistle   *spider*

(3)   [wado]   [wɪdo]   [bado]   [bʌdo]

water   *whistle*   *spider*   *butter*

Notice that the selection of processes is totally determined by the interest in eliminating the homonyms. For example, we could have selected the process of vocalization (i.e. [l], [r] → [o]) to eliminate. This, however, would no thave affected the homonymy at all. Instead the processes of alveolar assimilation (*1*), glide stopping (*2*), and vowel neutralization would be eliminated. The selection of processes will of course vary for different forms and different children. The goal to eliminate homonyms, however, is constant.

6.33   Contrasts within the child's system

While establishing contrasts by stabilizing pronunciation and eliminating homonyms works on a word-to-word basis, the general goal of establishing new contrasts takes the child's entire system into account. The former two methods are the result of examining the child's sample for particularly troublesome words. The latter reflects a more general analysis of the child's system of contrasts. Teaching by this method will subsequently include a wide variety of words, since the contrasting sounds, rather than the words, are the focus.

This can be first exemplified by looking at the development of the vowel system. Suppose that a child's system is very primitive and all vowels are neutralized to [a], or some phonetic alternative such as [ə]. One approach would be to start randomly training the English vowel system. This, however, would be an unprincipled approach in that it does not consider the fact that learning is gradual (*cf.* section 6.42), nor that the child builds up contrasts in a systematic way. A principled approach, however, would be to build up gradually a system of contrasts.

A useful guide for the selection of contrasts is the work of Jakobson (1968), although his suggestions only deal with the earliest contrasts. For vowels, he has noted that the first contrast is between [a] and a high vowel, either [i] or [u]. The selection of one or the other for work in therapy could depend on the individual child. Some may show occasional use of one or the other, which would then be the best choice. The next step is the basic three vowel system—[i], [a], [u]. Although Jakobson concentrates only on these three, there is some evidence that [e] and [o] are the next to appear (Velten 1943). Since vowels develop rapidly in normal children's speech, there is relatively little detailed information on vowel development. One further point that can be mentioned, however, is that the tense-lax distinction seems to appear after the tense vowels are used, i.e. [i], [e], [o], [u]. The following are some examples from Aaron's speech which suggest that lax vowels will still undergo vowel neutralization even when tense vowels are used:

	Tense		Lax
i	*bee* [bi], *tea* [ti]	ɪ	*window* [dʌdo], *stick* [sʌk]
e	*paper* [peto], *snake* [sek]	ɛ	*bed* [tʌt], *desk* [sʌk]
u	*boot* [put], *shoe* [sup]	ʊ	*book* [bʌk], *foot* [pat]
o	*rope* [wop], *stove* [dov]	ɔ	*fork* [pak], *dog* [kak]

From all these observations one could then establish a plan of therapy for the hypothetical subject with [a] to build up a system of contrasts gradually. Table 38 shows what one such programme might look like. Since a child with a primitive vowel system is also usually a child with reduced syllables, these would be first established in monosyllables, CV and CVC, and then in syllables that do not carry primary stress.

Table 38 Some possible systems of vowel contrasts built up from the basic vowel /a/

Two-vowel system	a—i	(or)	a—u			
Three-vowel system	i		u			
			a			
Four-vowel system	i		u			
	e	a				
Five-vowel system	i		u			
	e		o			
			a			
Six-vowel system	i		u			
	e		o			
	æ	a				
Lax vowels and diphthongs	i–ɪ		u–ʊ	ay		
	e–ɛ		o–ɔ	aw	oy	
	æ	a				

The suggestion that the establishment of contrasts is an important part of therapy has appeared before in the literature, particularly in Haas 1963 and Weber 1970. Since deviant children usually have more problems with consonants than vowels, consonant contrasts have been the focus of these works. Kevin, the child studied by Haas, used the following system of word initial consonant contrasts:

p   t
m   n
w   s

To increase this system, Haas suggests the following steps:

(*1*)   add a t–k contrast
(*2*)   add a b–d contrast
(*3*)   add a d–g contrast
(*4*)   add simultaneously a t–f contrast
                               f–s contrast
(*5*)   add voiced–voiceless contrast
p–b; t–d; k–g
(*6*)   add b–w–r and l–w–v;
          also s–θ–f and begin work with clusters.

He also states that final consonants should be worked on at all steps.

While these steps provide one way that contrastive training may proceed, it is not clear that these are necessarily the best to choose. The first step is a reasonable choice, in that Jakobson has argued that the stop consonants develop from a [p]–[t] contrast to a [p], [t], [k] one. Establishing the contrast with [k] involves the elimination of fronting, showing the interaction between processes and contrasts. The goal of establishing *contrasts* provides a principled way of deciding on what process to eliminate first. The selection of [k] to teach, however, also makes the assumption that it is one that is prior to other possible contrasts. Unfortunately, this is difficult to determine since many factors are involved, particularly the fact that we simply do not know with certainty the order of acquisition. Consequently the selection process will have to be intuitive in many cases, and failure to establish one contrast will require the selection of another.

There is one way that the selection of contrasts could proceed. Below is an inventory of the earlier consonants that appear in children's speech, based more or less on the findings discussed in chapter 2.

p   t
b   d
f   s   h
w   y
m   n

If it is possible to speak of a basic set of consonants, a reduced system like Kevin's could be compared with the core system. Matching Kevin's, we get the following, with Kevin's contrasts circled:

	Labial	*Alveolar*	*Palatal*	*Velar*	*Glottal*
stop:	(p)	(t)			
	b	d			
fricative:	f	(s)			h
nasal:	(m)	(n)			
glide:	(w)		y		
liquid:		(none)			

Since the [p]–[t], [f]–[s] set shows only [f] lacking, this element would qualify as an early candidate. Next, the voiced series appears in order. Since Kevin does occasionally produce these, it shows that they may be developing as contrasts. This suggests at least two contrasts before the [t]–[k] one: (*1*) [p]–[f] and [s]–[f]; and (*2*) [p]–[b], and [t]–[d]. This would result in a different order than that given by Haas.

Notice also that once this is done, the attempt to eliminate fronting can be done more generally. Haas mentions only work on [k]. With the [p], [t], [b], [d] series established, fronting can be eliminated with work on both [k] and [g]. Since a voiced–voiceless series would be available, it makes it possible to attack the most general form of the process. These points can be condensed into two basic guidelines:

(*1*) establish contrasts that result in a system comparable to that used by young children, since the latter system presumably reflects some notion of order of difficulty; and

(*2*) proceed in a way that contrasts are established by eliminating processes in their most general form. The latter point of teaching a contrast through several segments of a process was emphasized by Weber (1970).

Ethel's sample (chapter 3) can be used to exemplify how the process of constructing some goals of therapy may proceed. In terms of instability, the word *pencil* is the most varied:

pencil	[peθ]	[pɛmp]
	[pɛmpʌ]	[pɛntɪ]
	[pɛmpa]	[pɛntʌ]

Based on her general processes, the underlying form of this for her is probably [pɛntʌ]. By stabilizing this particular form, several optional phonetic processes are eliminated. Once done, the more general processes that affect correct production are isolated:

pencil	[pɛnsl̩]	
	pɛnsə	vocalization
	pɛntə	stopping

Other unstable words would be stabilized in a similar way to isolate common processes. Regarding homonyms, there are relatively few in her speech. An example is [te] for *play, tail, take*. This could be eliminated by establishing a [p] in the first, and a final stop in the last. In Ethel's sample, the elimination of homonyms at this stage is not a major problem.

In terms of contrasts, the vowels appear to be used well, although there is the methodological problem of transcription as mentioned earlier. For consonants, the following initial system of contrasting sounds was isolated and compared against the core system of early speech (Ethel's forms are circled):

	Labial	Alveolar	Palatal	Velar	Glottal
stop	(p)	(t)			
	(b)	(d)			
fricative	f	s			(h)
nasal	(m)	n			
glide	(w)		y		
liquid		(none)			

It is useful to note which other sounds were also produced although their use was not stable. For Ethel, these are [l], [n], and [g].

Tables 15 and 16 present the major phonological processes of Ethel's speech. A set of goals designed to establish more contrasts will determine which of these processes can be eliminated first. The first gap in her system is [n], i.e. there is [b], [d], and [m]. The establishment of [n] will fill these contrasts and also eliminate the variation in her language between [m] and [n]. A similar gap is in the glides, and this suggests work on a [w]–[y] contrast. A next goal would be to establish at least one contrast in the two classes that have none, i.e. fricatives and liquids. Since [l] occasionally appears, it is a likely candidate for the liquid class. For fricatives, the choice would be between [f] and [s]. A glance at the stopping rule helps decide between these. The rule is [f], [s] → [t]. Since [s] is closer to [t] than [f], it should be easier to establish. A next step which would begin work beyond the core system is the establishing of [k] and [g] through the elimination of fronting.

Based on the above, a programme of teaching contrasts might look something like the one in table 39.

Table 39   A potential programme of therapy for word initial consonants for Ethel, based on the establishment of contrasts through the elimination of processes

Step	Contrast to establish	Process to eliminate
1	m—n	Avoidance of words with *n*
	d—n	Occasional substitution of n → m
2	w—y	Gliding: y → w
3	n—l	Liquid stopping: l → d
	d—l	
4	t—s	Stopping: t → s
5	p—f	(Based on success of step 4)
6	s—f	Stopping: f → t
7	t—k, d—g	Fronting: $\begin{bmatrix} k \\ g \end{bmatrix} \to \begin{bmatrix} t \\ d \end{bmatrix}$
8	k—g	

Besides initial consonants, medial and final contrasts will also need to be established. The analysis of Ethel II provided some facts that will assist in decisions on these. Table 16 shows that only two contrasts appear to be emerging in the medial position, these being [t]–[d], and [p]–[b]. These could constitute the first target of therapy in this position, in words like *pillow* [pɪda], [pɪta]. The latter shows that not only adult [b], [p], [t], [d] are involved, but also substitutions for other segments. Thus, part of establishing a contrast between [t]–[d] in Ethel's speech is to stabilize the substitution of [l] → [d]. Later, when [t]–[d] is established, one between [l]–[d] can begin to be established with the elimination of the liquid stopping process. [t], [p], [m], [n] are beginning to be used in the final position. These would be the first contrasts to establish in therapy. The elimination of the deletion of final consonants would be done systematically to establish these contrasts.

While the establishment of contrasts is within the child's own system, this system will come progressively closer to the adult one. The child with only one or two major phonological processes will only be lacking in one or two series of contrasts. In these cases, the teaching of contrasts is identical with the elimination of the process. In more serious cases, however, the number and generality of processes will be large. The establishment of contrasts in a systematic way will stimulate the child's ability to use speech contrastively as well as provide a rationale for the method of eliminating processes.

6.4 Some further issues

6.41 Deciding what to teach first

Most of the discussion so far has focused on *what* to teach, resulting in the conclusion that what needs to be taught is a progressive system of contrasts through the elimination of simplifying phonological processes. The *order* in which this is done is also important. In the earlier sections, suggestions have been made in this regard. This section will make these more explicit and evaluate some of the suggestions found in the literature.

The question can be stated like this: given that the child has a number of processes, which are to be eliminated first? It is not possible in most cases simply to say that all should be attempted simultaneously. In more severe cases this becomes impossible. Instead, certain ones have to be selected above others. Most of the studies that have combined linguistic analysis with therapy have avoided this issue (e.g. Compton 1970, Oller 1973). This may be because these studies were more concerned in pointing out that processes need to be considered instead of isolated sounds. Whatever the reason, however, few suggestions exist in this area.

An exception to this is the discussion contained in Edwards and Bernhardt 1973a. There the authors make three suggestions concerning the selection of processes for therapy. First, they feel that those processes resulting in the greatest unintelligibility should be selected. It is also noted that these may or may not be the more 'natural' processes used by the child. Unfortunately they do not define unintelligibility so that the determination of these is impressionistic. Secondly, if it is not possible to choose between several processes in this regard, first select those that are optional, i.e. those that only occur occasionally. Finally, if neither of the above holds, work first on those processes most characteristic of young children. Edwards and Bernhardt consider fronting, stopping, voicing changes, the deletion of final consonants, and labialization as the earliest processes.

These suggestions are certainly a step in the right direction. Since communication is the ultimate goal, the resolution of unintelligibility is an important consideration. Also, it is reasonable to expect that processes that occur only occasionally should be the easiest to eliminate. Consideration of the order of development in normal children is also worth while and it constitutes a major emphasis of this book. At the same time, however, these selections as stated are largely impressionistic. It is not easy to decide what leads to most unintelligibility, although intuition may help. Also, it is not always clear what is the acquisition process in normal children, since children may vary greatly from one another. Because of these problems, the Edwards and Bernhardt suggestions are somewhat vague and require a sophisticated knowledge of acquisition.

The emphasis on the establishment of contrasts and the acquisition of individual words makes the selections of processes more explicit. Edwards and Bernhardt examine the list of processes and try to determine from that list an order of treatment. The above approach, however, looks first at the child's actual *words* and his system of *contrasts*. It is on the basis of these and not the processes alone that the order is selected. The suggestions from the earlier section can be summarized as follows:

(*1*)   Stabilize the more highly unstable words in the child's speech. This will result in the use of one phonetic shape that isolates the more widely used processes. This suggestion reflects two aspects of the Edwards and Bernhardt suggestion. The first is that instability is the result of optional processes so that these are eliminated before less optional ones. Secondly, it deals directly with the question of intelligibility.

(*2*)   Determine those forms of the child's speech that result in the greatest homonymy. Reduce this homonymy by eliminating those processes that create it. Again, the issue is intelligibility.

(*3*)   Determine for vowels and consonants (in initial, medial, and final position) those sounds that are used contrastively in the child's speech. Compare these to those used by normal children at a comparable period. Establish new contrasts gradually on the basis of this comparison. (It is acknowledged here that determining the normal role of contrasts is not always easy or feasible.) Do this by eliminating those processes that stop the target contrasts from occurring.

The value of these procedures will vary from child to child. If a child has a very stable system (e.g. Joe), the first is of no importance. Also, if the child does not have widespread use of homonyms, the second is of little help. The third will be a problem when children show acquisition patterns that differ from what would be expected. The child R studied by Nice (1925), for example, had the following vowel system (*cf.* table 18):

u
o   ɾ
a

This differs from the development of vowels shown in table 38. In cases like these, one needs to use a basic knowledge of acquisition to improvise. R's system invites comparison to a basic five-vowel system:

    i   u
    e   o
        a

This indicates that a contrast with the two front vowels is in order. These are guidelines that will help in determining what contrasts need to be established first, but they are only as good as the analyst's insight into language development.

6.42   Degrees of correctness

It is often assumed without justification that the goal of therapy is correct pronunciation as compared with the adult model. For example, if Aaron says [dado] for *whistle*, the aim of therapy should be to get him to say [wɪsl]. For convenience I will refer to this assumption as the 'fell-swoop principle'. It claims that the transition from the child's word to the adult pronunciation should take place in one step.

As virtually every working language clinician knows, it is not possible to teach many words, and even sounds, in one fell swoop. Because of this, two basic approaches have occurred in therapy that deal with this fact and also maintain the fell-swoop principle. One is to teach sounds first either in isolation, or in nonsense syllables of a CV structure. The other is to avoid teaching both words and sounds that do not appear ready for fell-swoop acquisition. In Aaron's example, the teaching of word initial /w-/ would be in words the child can produce correctly if [w-] is correct, e.g. *we*, *way*, *white* etc. A word like *whistle* would be avoided, as would more difficult sounds. For example, if the child says [t] for /θ/, this might be avoided in therapy if correct production appeared impossible.

The fell-swoop principle, however, is unsound in several ways. First and perhaps foremost, it assumes incorrectly that the acquisition of phonology is an instantaneous process. All data collected on phonological development has shown that *acquisition is gradual*. A normal child does not learn the production of a sound in one step, but goes through several stages. To expect a deviant child to learn in one fell swoop is expecting more of him than one expects from the normal child. The fact that acquisition is gradual suggests that the teaching of a sound or word should be gradual. A change in the child's speech can be considered correct if it results in a closer approximation to the adult model.

Another inadequacy of this approach is the fact that it limits severely what a therapist can do at any one time. For example, if a child has the rule [f] → [t], and [f] cannot be established, then this sound will be abandoned. All words with [f] will remain highly unintelligible. At any one time, a number of a child's forms will be avoided because of considerations like these. Suppose, however, that the rule of [f] stopping could be altered to [f] → [s]. If the criteria of success is weakened to accept this, the words with [f] will at least be more intelligible than before, e.g. *foot* [tʊt] v. [sʊt]; *feather* [tɛtɾ] v. [sɛtɾ] etc. In cases like this, the intelligibility will increase.

One could respond that accepting a less than correct (by adult standards) production will result in frozen forms in the child's speech. That is, the child will keep this form once it is established and will resist future changes. There is not, however, any empirical evidence suggesting this. Certainly this is not a problem for the normal child who continues to advance. Also, therapy in syntax in deviant children has been proceeding in this fashion, teaching syntax in a stage by stage fashion (e.g. Miller and Yoder 1974), and the data to date suggest that this actually *increases* the rate of development (e.g. Fygetakis and Ingram 1973, Gottsleben, *et al.* 1974). This stands to reason, in that it is based on the assumption that a child will progress more rapidly to his next stage of development than to one several stages ahead. It is this assumption that is behind the approach advocated here, which could be referred to as the 'gradualness principle'.

While there is no data in support of the fell swoop principle, there are instances showing that it may actually retard development. A good example is provided in Compton 1970. He refers to Tom's form for *sock* as being [skak]. This, at first glance, appears to be a peculiar form. Upon closer examination, however, Compton found that the therapist had attempted to correct Tom's production of *sock* in one fell swoop to [sak]. The clinician said to the child, 'No, Tommy, say sssock.' Tommy ended up putting the [s] before the form he used. Compton notes: 'after a number of similar incidents, the child adopted [sk] into his speech as an "acceptable" pronunciation of /s/' (325). Thus, the use of this principle resulted in establishing an unusual and perhaps less intelligible production.

A different approach would have been to attack Tommy's production of *sock* as [kak] gradually. Notice that there are two processes involved:

/sak/	Adult form
tak	Stopping
kak	Velar assimilation

The first step would be to eliminate velar assimilation. In a gradual approach [tak] would have been accepted as correct for this step in the therapy. Only after velar assimilation was eliminated would the elimination of stopping be undertaken. The suggestion to teach gradually and accept intermediate improvements occasionally appears in the literature (e.g. Pollack and Rees 1972, West and Weber 1973).

One advantage of the gradualness principle is that it will probably lead to more rapid development. There is an important factor related to this. As the child's system becomes gradually more intelligible, his parents and siblings will find it easier to understand him. Gains in this aspect are crucial for encouraging communication in the home. Since therapy time is such a small part of a child's day, it is important to increase the child's opportunity for effective communication outside the clinic.

6.43   The role of discrimination training

Although the emphasis in this book has been on the production of phonology, there is also the question of including the perception or discrimination of sounds as part of diagnosis and therapy. Evidence from the study of normal children (*cf.* section 2.332) suggests that it develops gradually alongside productive use. The results from Shvachkin (1973 *cf.* table 4), Garnica 1973 and Edwards 1974 could be used as guidelines. The use of discrimination testing is a traditional part of language therapy. Templin (1957) tested for speech-sound discrimination as well as production. Witkin (1971) reflects this when he says that 'a test of speech sound discrimination is the most basic diagnostic tool of the speech therapist, and much remedial work centres on discrimination of various kinds' (cited in Rees 1973, 304–5).

Traditionally in therapy, a child learns to discriminate between two sounds before he or she is trained to produce them. Sometimes a great deal of discrimination therapy takes place before work on productive language begins. Eisenson 1972 (chapter 6), for example, is devoted entirely to a programme of discrimination in various degrees. At the end, he states: 'Children who can make these distinctions should be ready for the programmes in language production'(120). Others, however, have used this more moderately, teaching discrimination of certain contrasts before beginning work on them. Weber (1970) gave an articulation test to 18 subjects to isolate the deviant phonological processes. These were then tested by a discrimination test to see if faulty production occurred. Then, before articulation therapy began, discrimination training was undertaken. Subject M, for example (see table 33), had a general stopping process. Weber decided to teach the contrasts [t]–[s], [t]–[r], and [t]–[w]. To do this, M was first taught to discriminate between these. 'Once these contrasts were discriminated auditorily, he was then taught to produce them expressively' (140). This procedure of training discrimination before production is also suggested by Edwards and Bernhardt (1973a).

Although this procedure is commonly used by many clinicians, Rees (1973) has recently questioned its validity. Through an examination of various studies in the area of speech perception, she concludes that research is not clear in this regard. 'In sum, the evidence for an auditory factor at the basis of aphasic disorders is far from conclusive, and what positive results have been reported could well be interpreted to reveal what is already known—that these children have a language disorder' (308). Because of a lack of hard evidence that these children really have an auditory discrimination problem, she goes on to suggest that the use of discrimination training is very questionable. 'We must therefore question this diagnostic value of tests that purport to isolate these skills, as well as the therapeutic value of clinical procedures designed to improve them' (313).

Evidence that deviant children do not primarily have a perceptual problem challenges the widespread use of discrimination procedures. At the same time, there may be instances where individual children may have some·perceptual problems with specific sounds. Given this possibility, it may be unrealistic to abandon the use of discrimination altogether. Rather, it probably should be used occasionally when evidence suggests a perceptual confusion between sounds. A recent study by Salus and Salus (1974), for example, has suggested that fricatives are so difficult because of their perceptual properties. 'We believe that the acquisition and production of phonological entities presupposes their perception, and that the reason for the later acquisition of fricative consonants is that they are not discriminated by the immature nervous system' (156). Fricatives, then, may be more likely to result from a perceptual factor than other sounds. Certainly more research is needed into the value and limitations of discrimination training in therapy.

6.44   A note on the role of training syntax

A last point worthy of mention concerns the relationship between a child's phonological disorder and other general aspects of language breakdowns. In section 5.41 it was pointed out that some recent work suggests that a child with a phonological disability has a general language problem (e.g. Panagos 1974). This was also the suggestion at the end of the article by Rees (1973).

If this is so, it provides some speculation that the child's phonology can be improved by training or general language skills. Panagos (1974), in fact, suggests this approach. He states: 'In our own clinical experience at Kent State University we have had about a dozen severe articulation cases show spontaneous and rapid development of the sound system when their syntax was the focus of therapy' (30). Panagos is careful to point out that 'we do not have any experimental evidence that teaching syntax facilitates articulation development' (30). Because of this, it is not possible to eliminate the use of phonological therapy. It is an interesting area of research, however, and suggests that one day perhaps syntactic training will also be an important part of therapy directed towards resolving a child's phonological disorders.

7

Recent developments

7.0 Introduction

The previous six chapters have examined in some detail the major aspects of the study of phonological disability. In this closing chapter, I turn to a general discussion of some of the developments which have taken place since the original publication of the text in 1976. For the sake of simplicity, this will be done by denoting a section corresponding to each of the six previous chapters.

7.1 A Linguistic approach

Throughout the text, I have assumed that a sound knowledge of linguistics needs to underlie the study of phonological disability in children. This point was expressed in 1.3 in some detail, both in terms of linguistics in general and phonology in particular. At the same time, however, I did not explicity discuss what I mean by the term 'phonology'. This has proved to be unfortunate, in that I have found that this area of linguistics is sometimes misunderstood. I thus begin here with a general discussion of phonology. This discussion could be used in conjunction with Chapter 1 as an introduction to the study of phonological disability.

Phonology can be defined in the simplest way as the study of the sound patterns (or sound system) of a language. When discussing this area, I have found two general misunderstandings about what it means. One is that there is a difference between 'phonology' and 'language', e.g. "do you study phonology or language?". Within linguistics, however, language is normally treated as consisting of three core areas or components:

> syntax — the study of sentence structure
> semantics — the study of meaning
> phonology — the study of the sound system

Within this view, phonology is not distinct from language, but a part of it.

A second misunderstanding of phonology is that it is equivalent to articulation or speech. Phonology, however, is much more than just the study of speech sounds. We can see this by extending our definition of phonology:

> **Phonology** is the study of the way speech sounds are organized and represented in the mind.

This definition requires a distinction between 1. the articulation of speech sounds, and 2. their mental representation. We usually speak of this in terms of two distinct kinds of 'representations':

1. phonetic representation — how they are articulated
2. underlying representation — how they are stored in the mind.

A fundamental difference between these two is that the underlying (mental representation) consists of just those aspects of sound structure which are *nonredundant*, i.e. predictable by rule. We can show this by looking at the word 'pad', which has the phonetic representation of [pʰæːd̥]. Among its phonetic characteristics are aspiration of thé initial stop, the length of the vowel, and the fact that the final consonant is partially devoiced. All of these aspects are predictable by rule, and therefore not part of the underlying representation, which is /pæd/. These three segments or 'phonemes', however, i.e. /p/ /æ/ /d/, have to be represented because changes in them result in changes in meaning, e.g. p → b 'bad', æ → /a/ 'pod', or d → /t/ 'pat'.

We can now further define phonology as the study of the following three aspects:

1. the nature of the underlying representations,
2. the nature of the phonetic representations,
3. the rules which map between the two above.

The mapping between the underlying and phonetic representations is called a *derivation*. The derivation of our example 'pad' would thus be as follows:

EXAMPLE   /p   æ   d/
          pʰ   Aspiration
                   æ: Vowel lengthening
                       d̥   Final partial devoicing
          [pʰæd̥]

When linguists study the underlying representations in a language, they look at two aspects. One of these is a *set of phonotactic constraints*, i.e. restrictions on what can combine with what. For example, English has a phonotactic constraint against the following two clusters at the beginning of a syllable, *tl, *pw. The second aspect is the *phonemic inventory*, i.e. the distinctive sounds in the language. For English, we generally recognize the following consonantal and vocalic phonemes (also see Notation section at the beginning of the book):

Consonants:

p		t	č (chip)	k
b		d	ǰ (jeep)	g
m		n		- ŋ (sing)
f	(thing)	s	ʃ (shoe)	h-
v	(the)	z	- ȝ (rouge)	
		l		
		r		
w		·y		

Vowels:	i	(see)		u	(Sue)
	I	(sit)	(cut)	ʊ	(book)
	e	(say)		o	(boat)
	ɛ	(set)		ɔ	(bought)
	æ	(sat)	ɑ (cot)	Dipthongs ɑy (eye) ɔy (boy)	

While we discuss phonemes as units unto themselves, they can be further broken down into their individual *distinctive features*. For example, the phonemes /p/ and /f/ can be divided into features such as the following:

/p/	/f/
[+stop]	[–stop]
[+labial]	[+labial]
[+obstruent]	[+obstruent]

Linguists have not yet reached a consensus on the proper set of distinctive features to be used in describing phonemes, although the set suggested in Chomsky and Halle (1968) are still in common use. The features are important because they help us see general patterns.

The rules which map underlying representations into phonetic ones are referred to as *phonological rules* or *processes*. They are commonly written by indicating the features which are involved. For example, a rule which devoices final consonants as in German can be stated in the following way:

final devoicing

b		p		
d	→	t	rule	[+stop] → [–voice] ##
g		k		

Linguistics is a field constantly undergoing change in its attempts to construct a phonological theory. in 1.21, I mention that two popular theories in 1976 were *generative phonology* and *natural phonology*. The former is marked by an interest in capturing phonological rules through the use of features much in the way shown above. The latter attempts to build upon generative phonology by restricting the set of possible rules to those which follow from the properties of the human auditory/ articulatory system. Since the latter theory is based upon a simultaneous desire to account for patterns in child language, it has been heavily used in the text, especially Chapter 2.

There have been some subsequent developments since the original text which deserve comment in regard to the issue of phonological theory. One is that the proposal of 'phonological processes' has created a band-wagon effect of sorts in the area of phonological disability. This has been unfortunate in some cases because it has resulted in the production of lists of processes with little effort for their justification. Also, the research into natural phonology has been quite limited. The result of these two trends is that we know little more about what constitutes the set of natural processes now than we did 12 years ago. Another consequence of the concentration upon processes is that less work has been done on the study of children's underlying representations. As I will point out below, this, in fact, is probably the most fruitful aspect under investigation today.

Another major development has been an evolution of sorts in phonological theory. This is the emergence of a new view of phonology which has been referred to in many different ways, but which I will call *nonlinear phonology*. This approach differs rather dramatically from previous theories by dividing up how aspects of underlying representations are internally structured. Most generally, different features are placed on different levels or tiers. The advantage of this is that rules such as assimilation can be very simply described as the result of a feature moving along its tier.

For example, take the child form of [gak] for 'dog' where the first consonant has assimilated to the second. Nonlinear phonology would describe this in the following way. First, there is a level where timing units such as Cs (for consonants) and Vs (for vowels) are represented. Below this is a melodic level where distinctive features are hierarchically ordered, such as below:

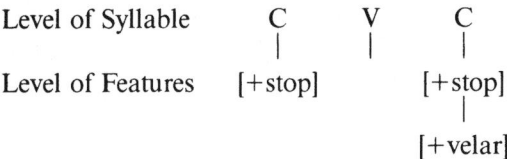

The child in this case only has the feature [+velar] for the second consonant but not for the first. This feature then spreads along its tier to the first consonant. It does not affect the vowel because vowels will never be specified for this feature.

The specifics of nonlinear phonology are currently being developed in the linguistic literature. Also, it has barely begun to be applied to language acquisition. It has, however, aspects which make it attractive as an account of phonological acquisition. Particularly, it is concerned with the universal set of features and exactly how they may be structured. I suspect that it will become the dominant theory in acquisition research for the next several years.

7.2 Phonological acquisition in normal children

Chapter 2 outlines in some detail several findings about how normal children acquire a phonological system. Much of that discussion, however, is descriptive, i.e. outlining milestones of phonological acquisition. The next step is to identify among all the various facts of acquisition those which in particular are going to play a significant role in our theory of acquisition.

The text mentions attempts to explain phonological acquisition by researchers such as Stampe and Jakobson, but the situation is such that we still do not have an accepted theory of phonological acquisition. This situation, however, is not a reason for despair. We can still have a good idea of how acquisition proceeds by establishing a basic set of assumptions based on what we know to date. Below I give 11 assumptions about normal acquisition which I feel will underlie any serious theory of phonological acquisition:

1. Research on infant speech perception has found that infants are remarkably good at identifying the acoustic characteristics of speech sounds. Their acoustic representations, therefore, should be reasonably complete.

2. When children acquire their 50th word in production around 1;6, they have a much larger receptive vocabulary, around 250 words. The latter vocabulary is sufficiently large to suggest that phonological organization has begun.

3. Given the discrepancy between spoken and receptive vocabularies just mentioned, spoken vocabulary should be considered a conservative estimate of the child's phonology.

4. Children show a word spurt around 1;6. This milestone suggests that a significant change in the child's phonological organization has taken place.

5. My research suggests that children begin phonological organization from the acquisition of their first words. This early system, as shown in Chapter 2, is restricted to a small number of syllable shapes and phonological features.

6. Phonological contrasts often first enter the child's system in a very restricted way. For example, a child who has the consonants /p/, /b/, /t/, /k/, and /b/, has only acquired the voicing contrast for the labial position.

7. Recent research by Schwartz and Leonard (1982) has shown that children select certain sounds of adult words and avoid others. This suggests a much more developed phonology of the receptive vocabulary.

8. Children's first substitutions are at first restricted in the same way as contrasts are as stated in 6. For example, a child might first use [b] for adult words beginning with /b/, and then spread its use to words beginning with /p/ and /f/.

9. My recent research suggests that children show three patterns of sound development over the first months of word acquisition — (1) lexical, i.e. a sound only found in a single word, (2) gradual, i.e. a sound spreading gradually to more and more words and (3) abrupt, i.e. a sound shows a sudden occurrence in several words. These different patterns need to be taken into consideration when we decide whether a sound is or is not part of the child's system.

10. Research reported in Pye, Ingram and List (1987) indicates that children acquire a 'basic' set of sounds first, and that this basic set will vary from language to language. This suggests that phonologically more prominent sounds are acquired before less prominent ones.

11. Development after the word spurt appears to be primarily the spreading of the 'basic' sounds into new combinations, rather than the addition of new sounds.

A general feeling for the kinds of development discussed above can be obtained by examining one child's acquisition of English initial consonants. Below I give a chart which shows how T, originally studied in Ferguson and Farwell (1975), acquired her initial consonants. I first show her phonetic inventory, and then the adult sounds they occurred for. Parentheses indicate those sounds which only appeared in a single word. Asterisks indicate sounds which appeared in three or more words. All other sounds occurred in two words.

Session Phonetic Inventory

	[m	n	b	d	p	t	k	s	ʃ	h	w]
1				d							
2				d			(k)			(h)	
3	(m)			*d						h	
4	(m)		b	*d		(t)			(ʃ)	(h)	
5	(m)		b	*d		(t)		s	(ʃ)		(w)
6	(m)	(n)	*b	d	*p	t		s	ʃ	(h)	(w)
7	m	(n)	*b	d	*p	*t	(k)		(ʃ)	(h)	w
8	(m)	(n)	*b			*t	(k)		ʃ	(h)	w
9	(m)	(n)	*b	d	*p	*t	k	s	(ʃ)	(h)	w

Session Matches and Substitutions

	/m	n	b	d	p	t	k	s	č		h	w	y	r/
1				d				(h)						
2				d				(h)			(?)			
3	(m)		(d)	d		(t)		(h)	(g)		(h)			
4	(m)		b	d				(ʃ)	(ʃ)		(h)			
5	(m)		b	d				s	(ʃ)		(?)			(w)
6	(m)	(n)	b	d	p	(t)		s	(ʃ)		(h)		(y)	(w)
7	m	(n)	b	d	p	t	(k)	(ʃ)	(ʃ)	(t)	(h)	(w)	(y)	(w)
8	(m)	(n)	b	d	p	t	(T)	ʃ	(ʃ)	(t)	(h)	(w)	(y)	(w)
9	(m)	(n)	b	d	p	t	k	s	(ʃ)	(t)	(h)	(w)	(y)	(b)

We can see that T acquired her initial consonants in six steps:

1. |d|
2. |b| |d|
3. |b| |d| |s|
4. |b| |d|
   |p|
   |s|
5. |b| |d|
   |p| |t|
   |s|
6. |b| |d|
   |p| |t| |k|
   |s|

These six steps show the gradual spread of features mentioned in *observation 6*. For example, [voice] seems to be tied to T's first acquiring a new place feature. After |b| is acquired, T then acquires |p|. The new voice distinction, however, is not immediately spread to |d|. Also notice that the velar position is added as |k| without a voiced counterpart. T's previous pattern suggests that |g| will be next, and indeed, one [g] does occur in the last session.

T's data also indicates the *three patterns of emergence* mentioned in observation 9.

The nasals and [h] show a lexical pattern across the sessions. They are used, but only in single forms. [m], for example, was occurring in 'mommy' while [n] was used in 'no'. At the other extreme, [p] indicates the abrupt pattern of onset. At session VI, she suddenly used [p] in several words, while it was never used before this session. Most other sounds show a gradual pattern, becoming more frequent in each subsequent session.

The sounds that T has at session IX are actually a subset of the basic set usually acquired by English children. Below I give the basic set for English, based on Ingram (1981). Also, I compare these to the basic set found in Pye, Ingram and List (1987) for Quiché, a Guatamalan language. This indicates how different the basic sets can be, and the importance of how phonologically prominent a sound is.

English			Quiché				
m	n		m	n			
b	d	g	p	t	č	k	ʔ
p	t	k				x	
f	s	h					
w			w				
				1			

It is particularly interesting to look at [s], [1], and [č]. While English has [1] and [č], they are not normally among the first speech sounds acquired in English. In Quiché, however, they are not only early, but also are two of the most frequently used sounds. At the same time [s], which occurs in Quiché, is not a particular early sound for Quiché children. In Pye, Ingram and List, we use such differences to emphasize how children are sensitive to lanaguage specific differences at a very early point of phonological acquisition.

7.3 Phonological analysis

The phonological analysis of children's language has been a highly researched area in the years since 1976. Attempts to do this can be found in Weiner (1979), Shriberg and Kwiatkowski (1980), Hodson and Paden (1983), and Khan (1986). Many of these, however, have concentrated only exclusively on phonological processes. As mentioned above, however, phonological analysis needs to go beyond looking just at these. Chapter 3 of this text has emphasized that analysis includes determining also the child's phonetic inventory, substitution patterns, and phonological features. This approach has been developed further in Ingram (1981), and also from a different perspective in Grunwell (1985).

The most recent suggestions of mine in this regard are found in Ingram (1989). There I suggest the following three steps to phonological analysis:

1. Determination of the phonetic inventory
2. Determination of the child's matches and substitutions
3. Determination of the child's phonological oppositions

The result of this kind of analysis has been presented just above in a simplified form for the data from T. First, I found out the initial consonants which she used, along with some information about their frequency. The latter is important because we do not want to claim a child has acquired something when it is infrequent. Next, I looked at the sounds in English for which these sounds were used. For example, [t] was used correctly for /t/ and also a substitution for /č/. Likewise [s] and [ʃ] seemed to be used for both /s/ and /ʃ/, suggesting that these two adult sounds are not yet being distinguished.

The third step, the determination of the child's phonological oppositions, is the most difficult inventory. Above I did this in a simple fashion by focussing on the phonetic one. This led to the six steps which I discussed. This procedure will often provide a sufficient insight. For more serious research and theoretical purposes, however, a more detailed effort is needed. Ingram (1988) discusses some of the issues which are at stake as well as some suggestions for dealing with them.

The completion of a comprehensive phonological analysis, particularly along the lines of those in Chapter 3, Ingram (1981, 1989), and Grunwell (1985), can be a time consuming task. This is a serious concern of language clinicians who often do not have the time for such extensive analyses. To help this problem, there are efforts underway to develop personal computer programs which do much of this work. One such program is outlined in Pye and Ingram (1988).

7.4   Methodology

Chapter 4 provides a series of suggestions on the elicitation and transcription of phonological samples. This basic discussion is as relevant now as when it was written. Shriberg and Kwiatkowski (1981) have recently pointed out a rather serious problem with most articulation tests. They demonstrate that most of such tests typically use words which are relatively complex when compared with the words children usually use in their spontaneous speech. In other words, the words used put the child at a disadvantage. This is also true of more recent suggestions for word lists to elicit. For example, the suggested words in Hodson and Paden (1983) contain a very high number of consonant clusters. Shriberg and Kwiatkowski's suggestion is to avoid articulation tests altogether and rely exclusively on spontaneous samples.

7.5   The nature of deviant phonology

An issue which is treated at some length in Chapter 5 is the extent to which we can say that children with a phonological disorder are different from normal children. Chapter 5 outlines some of the issues and reviews some of the suggestions in the literature. The conclusion drawn is that the deviant child does in many cases look different because early patterns of substitution may persist along with later patterns to form a higher level of unintelligibility than that usually found in normal children.

I have recently reassessed this topic in two recent works (Ingram 1987a, 1987b). Here I will attempt to summarize the main points of those articles. First I observed that the study of categories of phonological disorders in children has been primarily motivated by two goals:

1. to place variation between children with phonological disorders into a general theory of phonological delay;
2. to provide a diagnosis for their proper assessment and remediation.

I will provide here a discussion of the first goal. See Ingram (1987a) for a treatment of the second one.

In order to establish a theory of phonological disorders, we need all of the following:

1. The development of a phonological theory;
2. The development of a theory of phonological acquisition;
3. The development of a theory of phonological disorders.

That is, we will need an already established phonological theory and a theory of normal acquisition.

I have already mentioned that phonological theory is undergoing rapid change, with the development of nonlinear phonology. This theory, however, is hardly at a point where its dimensions are well established. Further, I have mentioned that we still lack a theory of normal acquisition. The most likely candidates are:

1. Jakobson's long discussed universalist theory (1968);
2. Stampe's natural phonology (1969), and
3. the recent cognitive theory that has come out of Stanford University (Macken and Ferguson 1983). This theory is also discussed in Stoel-Gammon and Dunn (1985).

These theories have helped to sharpen the issues in the debate, but they have hardly solved the problem. Only one of these, Stampe's natural phonology, is even tied directly to a phonological theory. The Stanford theory emphasizes variation to such a degree that it is not even clear what general patterns of acquisition it predicts, if any. My own criticism of this approach is found in Goad and Ingram (1988). Given this situation, it is unlikely that we can have much hope at this time to come up with a well defined linguistic theory of disorders.

There are, however, two general issues which can be researched to establish some information about phonological disorders. One is to examine data to see if children's phonological patterns are reflecting an articulatory or linguistic problem. Chapter 5 has taken the position that their problems are primarily linguistic in nature. This position has been forcefully argued subsequently in Grunwell (1981).

A second line of research concerns looking at data from phonologically disordered children to see if they show patterns not found in normal children. Since 1976, our data base in the field has increased, aided by the publication of the actual data from seven children in Grunwell (1981). Leonard (1985) has provided a very nice review of a wide range of these data. These works as well as others have suggested that, as concluded in Chapter 5, deviant children are different in some significant way.

While this conclusion seems to have a consensus of sorts, there is a serious problem with it. The problem is that we can only be confident in concluding that deviant children are different, if we have a theory of acquisition which captures the range of variation between normal children. No such theory, however, currently exists. I think that our initial interest in concluding differences for children with phonological disorders resulted from the striking example of a small number of peculiar cases. As I point out in Ingram (1987b), however, there are quite a range of such cases also found with so-called normal children. Here are just a few examples:

a. Joan Velten (Velten 1943) shortened certain vowels when they occurred in contexts in English where they aré normally lengthened, and lengthened others which appeared in contexts where they are normally shortened;

b. Daniel Menn (Menn 1971) clearly showed superior acquisition of final consonants over initial ones.

c. A Smith (Smith 1973) deleted initial /s-/ at one stage, but not if it had already assimilated to a following velar consonant;

d. P Waterson (Waterson 1971) replaced a number of English initial consonants with a palatal nasal, and others with a bilabial fricative, a non-English speech sound.

My conclusion, then, is that we have yet to establish what normal children may or may not be able to do, and therefore cannot claim unique differences for disordered children.

There is, however, a problem for this conclusion. As pointed out by Leonard (1985), there are several case studies of children with phonological disorders where patterns have occurred which seem unlikely to be found with normal children. Some examples are;

a. a child who made ingressve /s/'s (Ingram and Terselic 1983);

b. a child who produced final nasal snorts (Edwards and Bernhardt 1973);

c. a child whose first fricatives were dental (Weiner 1981).

The position I have taken, therefore, cannot be maintained unless similar cases can be found with normal children.

The response to such cases in Ingram (1987a, 1987b) is to deal with them through two proposals. The first is a very simple hypothesis about the relation between vocabulary growth and phonological proficiency:

A Hypothesis about Phonological Deviance

'The extent of a child's phonological deviance is the consequence of an inverse relation between his stage of phonological acquisition and the size of his vocabulary.'

This proposal predicts that a phonologically disordered child is one who is at a very early stage of phonological development with a vocabulary which is much larger than that normally found.

There are at least two ways in which this situation could manifest itself. One is through the occurrence of unusual and pervasive substitutions. Normal children will often show such processes during the acquisition of their first fifty words. The child T referred to above, for example, showed the use of a palatal fricative as a substitute for both the initial alveolar /s-/ and palato-alveolar / -/. This would have appeared deviant if it had persisted.

The other way this could occur is through the occurrence of homonymy. In Chapter 5, for example, I have suggested that extensive homonymy characterizes the language of at least some children with phonological disorders. More recently, I have examined the development of homonymy in three children (Ingram 1985). I found that two of them showed increases in their phonetic inventories along with vocabulary growth. The other, however, the famous Hildegard Leopold, showed little change in her phonetic inventory while the vocabulary increased into the hundreds. The result was that her homonymy measure soared instead of decreased as it did for the other two children.

One particular feature about this hypothesis is that it does away to an extent with the distinction between normal children and children with phonological disorders altogether. Instead, all children will fall along a continuum regarding the relation between phonological stage and vocabulary. Hildegard therefore was phonologically deviant for the months described above.

Despite this proposal, there are a few cases left which still look rather peculiar. Interestingly, most of these involve the production of fricatives. My proposal for these remaining cases is that they may have been clinically induced through traditional procedures of therapy. This should not be surprising if one looks at the assumptions of the traditional method. It concentrates on the production of a single sound, with the hope of rapid improvement. If the child is under such pressure but not yet capable of making the appropriate change, he may attempt to do just about anything to show some change.

An example of such an effect was discussed earlier in Chapter 5. Compton (1970) reports a case of a child who produced [sk] for /s/, a peculiar substitute which Compton traced back to the child's therapy program. The child in question was producing /s/ in "sock" as [k] due to assimilation to the following velar. The attempts to get "sock" correct led to the imposition of the new [s] onto the previous substitute [k].

7.6 On remediation

Chapter 6 emphasizes two basic aspects of phonological remediation — 1. the elimination of phonological processes, and 2. the establishment of phonological contrasts. The former addresses the mapping between underlying and phonetic representations, while the latter deals with underlying representations directly. This is done after careful analysis of the child's system along the lines discussed above and in Chapter 3. Importantly, each intervention situation will need to be adapted to the individual characteristics of the child.

Chapter 6 does not make detailed suggestions on the step by step fashion in which remediation might proceed. A logical approach to this issue is to view the general findings on phonological acquisition in normal children and base a remedial approach upon them. In Ingram (1987a) I outline four such findings which I feel are particularly important for the development of a remedial program.

Each is repeated below, followed by its implications for therapy:

1. Children's receptive development consistently is in advance of their production. Phonologically, children show perception of phonemic oppositions that may not show up in their production until months later.

IMPLICATION: Initiate intervention with a concentration on developing receptive knowledge. Do not expect correct production to occur simultaneously with receptive development.

2. Children acquire a linguistic system, not specific rules. Phonologically, children are developing a system of phonological oppositions, not specific sounds.

IMPLICATION: Present the child with linguistic material which demonstrates a sound's role in the linguistic system. For example, if a child does not have /s-/, present the child with words with /s-/ which are similar to other words in his system with other sounds, e.g. 'six' vs 'fix' vs 'mix'. Secondly, systematically present a range of speech sounds, not just one.

3. Language acquisition is gradual. That is, the internalization of the linguistic system takes time. It involves the representation of the phonological form of words in the mind and the ability to retrieve that information and translate it into speech production. Not surprisingly, the consequence is that this process takes several months and predicts that neither receptive nor productive development is instantaneous.

IMPLICATION: Allow time for the child to develop a phonological unit into his receptive knowledge. Do not expect receptive knowledge, nor later production, to be established instantaneously.

4. Language acquisition is sensitive to linguistic input. Recent research on crosslinguistic phonological acquisition indicates that the first sounds of children are more influenced by their linguistic prominence in the language than by their assumed articulatory difficulty (c.f. Pye, Ingram and List 1987).

IMPLICATION: The phonological information presented to the child should be robust enough to establish its importance in the system. For example, teaching the child a series of words with /s-/ will requires the number of words to be sufficiently large as to demonstrate its linguistic value.

A recent approach to remediation which assumes several of these findings in its program can be found in Hodson and Paden (1983). In Ingram (1986), I discuss in some detail the rationale which underlies their program. Here I will briefly provide a general summary.

Calling their program a 'cyclical' approach, Hodson and Paden begin with an assessment of the child's system. This assessment will form the basis of the rest of the therapy. It should identify a range of phonemes which the child needs to acquire, and the patterns of substitution which are used in their place. Normally, six to twelve sounds are selected for direct intervention.

Intervention begins with what is referred to as the first cycle. Each cycle will last approximately 12 weeks, and several cycles may be needed. This cycle has the following features:

a. One sound is selected each week for therapy;
b. Two word lists are created with this target sound. One has 15 words and the other 5 words. For example, the latter list for word initial /p/ might be 'pot', 'pan', 'pen', 'peach', 'pole'.
c. The session begins with the clinician reading the 15 word list to the child.
d. The session then proceeds with the clinician presenting the words in a variety of tasks during the session. The child is not forced to pronounce the words correctly.
e. The word list is read once more at the end of the session.
f. The parents are asked to read the five word list to the child each day for the rest of the week.
g. Importantly, one does not expect articulatory progress in the first cycle.

The first cycle allows a range of speech sounds to be presented to the child over a reasonable length of time. The word lists enable the child to see the phonological function of each sound.

After the first cycle, there is a reassessment to see if progress has been made, and new target sounds are selected, if such is the case. Then, the second cycle proceeds in a similar fashion to the first. Progress, however, should be more noticeable after this and subsequent cycles.

Hodson and Paden have found the cyclical approach to be highly effective in helping children with phonological problems. It addresses both of the goals discussed in Chapter 6, i.e. it eliminates phonological processes and establishes new phonological contrasts. As mentioned in Ingram (1986), the approach still lacks theoretical justification for some of its assumptions. Nonetheless, it has proven to be an effective approach with an underlying rationale based on findings from normal language acquisition.

References

Abbreviations:

J. Educ. Psych.	*Journal of Educational Psychology*
J. Educ. Res.	*Journal of Educational Research*
JSHD	*Journal of Speech and Hearing Disorders*
JSHR	*Journal of Speech and Hearing Research*
PCLS	*Papers from the Chicago Linguistic Society*
Ped. Sem.	*Pedagogical Seminary*
PRCLD	*Papers and Reports on Child Language Development* (Stanford University)

ADAMS, N. 1972: Unpublished phonological diary of son Philip from 1;7 to 2;3.

APPLEGATE, J. 1961: Phonological rules of a subdialect of English. *Word* **17**, 186–93.

ATKINSON-KING, K. 1973: *Children's acquisition of phonological stress contrasts*. UCLA Working Papers in Phonetics **25**.

BANGS, J. 1942; A clinical analysis of the articulatory defects of the feebleminded. *JSHD* **7**, 343–56.

BATEMAN, W. 1916: The language status of three children at the same ages. *Ped. Sem.* **23**, 211–40.

BERKO, J. 1958: The child's learning of English morphology. *Word* **14**, 150–77.

BERKO, J. and BROWN, R. 1960: Psycholinguistic research methods. In P. Mussen (ed.), *Handbook of research methods in child development*. New York: Wiley.

BLOUNT, B. 1970: The pre-linguistic systems of Luo children. *Anthropological Linguistics* **12**, 326–42.

BODINE, A. 1974: A phonological analysis of the speech of two Mongoloid (Down's Syndrome) boys. *Anthrop. Linguistics* **16**, 1, 1–24.

BRAINE, M. 1971: The acquisition of language in infant and child. In C.E. Reed (ed.), *The learning of language*. New York: Appleton-Century-Crofts.

BROWN, R. 1973: *A first language*. Cambridge, Mass.: Harvard University Press.

BUSH, C. *et al.* 1973: On specifying a system for transcribing consonants in child language: a working paper with examples from American English and Mexican Spanish. Unpublished paper, Child Language Project, Stanford University.

BYRNE, M.C., SHELTON, R.L., DIETRICH, W.M. 1961: Articulatory skill, physical management, and classification of children with cleft palates. *JSHD* **26**, 326–33.

BZOCH, K.R. 1965: Articulation proficiency and error patterns of preschool cleft palate and normal children. *Cleft Palate Journal* **2**, 340–49.

CALVERT, D.R. 1962: Speech sound duration and the surd-sonant error. *Volta Review* **64**, 401–2.

CARR, J. 1953: An investigation of the spontaneous speech sounds of five-year-old deaf-born children. *JSHD* **18**, 22–9.

CARTER, E.T. and BUCK, M. 1958: Prognostic testing for functional articulation disorders among children in the first grade. *JSHD* **23**, 124–33.

CHOMSKY, C. 1969: *The acquisition of syntax in children from five to ten*. Cambridge, Mass.: MIT Press.

CHOMSKY, N. 1957: *Syntactic structures*. The Hague: Mouton.

CHOMSKY, N. and HALLE, M. 1968; *The sound pattern of English*. New York: Harper & Row.

COMPTON, A.J. 1970: Generative studies of children's phonological disorders. *JSHD* **35**, 315-39.

— 1975: Generative studies of children's phonological disorders: a strategy of therapy. In S. Singh (ed.), *Measurement in Hearing, Speech and Language*. Baltimore: University Park Press.

CROCKER, J.R. 1969: A phonological model of children's articulation competence. *JSHD* **34**, 203-13.

CRYSTAL, D. 1971: *Linguistics*. Harmondsworth, Middx.: Penguin.

— 1972: The case of linguistics: a prognosis. *British J. of Disorders in Communication* **7**, 3-16.

CRYSTAL, D., FLETCHER, P. and GARMAN, M. Second edition, 1989: *The grammatical analysis of language disability: a procedure for assessment and remediation*. London: Cole and Whurr.

CURTISS, S., FROMKIN, V., KRASHEN, S., RIGLER, D. and RIGLER, M. 1974: The linguistic development of Genie. *Language* **50**, 528-54.

DANILOFF, R. and STEPHENS, M.I. 1974: Unpublished research reported at the Annual Convention of the American Speech and Hearing Association.

EDWARDS, M.L. 1973: The acquisition of liquids. In G. Drachman (ed.), *Working Papers in Linguistics* **15**, 1-54, Ohio State University.

— 1974: Perception and production in child phonology: the testing of four hypotheses. *Journal of Child Language* **1**, 205-19.

EDWARDS, M.L. and BERNHARDT, B. 1973a; Phonological analyses of the speech of four children with language disorders. Unpublished paper, Stanford University.

— 1973b: Twin speech as the sharing of a phonological system. Unpublished paper, Stanford University.

EDWARDS, M.L. and GARNICA, O. 1973; Patterns of variation in the repetition of utterances by young children. Unpublished paper, Stanford University.

EIMAS, P. 1974; Linguistic processing of speech by young infants. In Schiefelbusch and Lloyd, 55-73.

EISENSON, J. 1972: *Aphasia in children*. New York: Harper & Row.

FAIRBANKS, G. 1940: *Voice and articulation drillbook*. New York: Harper & Row.

FAIRCLOTH, M.A. and FAIRCLOTH, S.R. 1970: An analysis of the articulatory speech defective child in connected and in isolated word responses. *JSHD* **35**, 51-61.

FERGUSON, C. 1968: *Contrastive analysis and language development*. Monograph series on language and linguistics **21**, 101-12, Georgetown University.

FERGUSON, C. and FARWELL, C. 1975: Words and sounds in early language acquisition: English initial consonants in the first 50 words. *Language* **51**. (Citation in text from version in *PRCLD* 1973, **6**, 1-61.)

FERGUSON, C. and GARNICA, O. 1975: Theories of phonological development. In E. Lenneberg and E. Lenneberg (eds.), *Foundations of language development*. UNESCO.

FERGUSON, C., PEIZER, D. and WEEKS, T. 1973: Model-and-replica phonological grammar of a child's first words. *Lingua* **31**, 35-65.

FLAVELL, J. 1963: *The developmental psychology of Jean Piaget*. New York: Van Nostrand.

FROMKIN, V. and RODMAN, R. 1974: *An introduction to language*. New York: Holt, Rinehart and Winston.

FRY, D.B. 1966: The development of the phonological system in the normal and deaf child. In F. Smith and G. Miller (eds.), *The genesis of language*, 187-206. Cambridge, Mass.: MIT Press.

FYGETAKIS, I. and INGRAM, D. 1973: Language rehabilitation and programmed conditioning: a case study. *Journal of Learning Disabilities* **6**, 60-4.

GARNICA, O. 1973: The development of phonemic speech perception. In T. Moore, 215-22.

GIMSON, A.C. 1970: *An introduction to the pronunciation of English*. Second edition, London: Edward Arnold.

GOAD, H. and INGRAM, D. 1988: Individual variation and its relevance to a theory of phonological acquisition. *Journal of Child Language* **14**, 419-32.

GOTTSLEBEN, R., TYACK, D. and BUSCHINI, G. 1974: Three cases in language training: applied linguistics. *JSHD* **39**, 213-24.

GREENLEE, M. 1973: Some observations on initial English consonant clusters in a child two to three years old. *PRCLD* **6**, 97-106.

— 1974: Interacting processes in the child's acquisition of stop-liquid clusters. *PRCLD* **7**, 85-100.

GRUNWELL, P. 1981: *The nature of phonological ability in children*. London: Academic Press.

— 1985: *Phonological assessment of child speech (PACS)*. San Diego: College Hill Press.

HAAS, W. 1963: Phonological analysis of a case of dyslalia. *JSHD* **28**, 239-46.

HAMP, E. 1974: Reduplications and monosyllables. *Journal of Child Language* **1**, 287.

HENDERSON, F. 1938: Objectivity and constancy of judgement in articulation testing. *J. Educ. Res.* **31**, 348-56.

HILLS, E.C. 1914: The speech of a child two years of age. *Dialect Notes* **4**, 84-100.

HINCKLEY, A. 1915; A case of retarded speech development, *Ped. Sem.* **22**, 121-46.

HODSON, B. and PADEN, E. 1983: *Targeting intelligible speech: a phonological approach to remediation*. College Hill Press: San Diego.

HUDGINS, C.V. 1934; A comparative study of the speech coordination of deaf and normal subjects. *Ped. Sem.* **44**, 3-48.

HUDGINS, C.V. and NUMBERS, F.C. 1942: *An investigation of the intelligibility of the speech of the deaf*. Genetic Psychology Monograph **25**, 289-392.

HUMPHREYS, M.W. 1880: A contribution to infantile linguistics. *Transactions of the American Philological Association* **11**, 5-17.

INGRAM, D. 1974a: Phonological rules in young children. *Journal of Child Language* **1**, 49-64.

— 1974b: Fronting in child phonology. *Journal of Child Language* **1**, 233-41.

— 1975a: The acquisition of fricatives and affricates in normal and linguistically deviant children. In A. Caramazza and E. Zuriff (eds.), *The acquisition and breakdown of language*. Baltimore: Johns Hopkins University Press.

— 1975b: *If and when transformations are acquired by children*. Monograph Series on Languages and Linguistics, Georgetown University **27**.

— 1975c: Surface contrast in phonology: evidence from children's speech. *Journal of Child Language* **2**, 287-92.

— 1981: *Procedures for the phonological analysis of children's language*. Baltimore, Md.: University Park Press.

— 1985: On children's homonyms. *Journal of Child Language* **12**, 671-80.

— 1986: Explanation and phonological remediation. *Child Language Teaching and Remediation* **2**, 1-29.

— 1987a: Categories of phonological disorder. *Proceedings of the First International Symposium on Specific Speech and Language Disorders in Children*. Surrey: Association for All Speech Impaired Children, 88-99.

— 1987b: Phonological impairment in children. Paper presented at the International Symposium entitled Language Acquisition and Language Impairment, Parma, Italy, June -46, 1987.

— 1988: Jakobson revisited: some evidence from the acquisition of Polish phonology. *Lingua* **75**, 55-82.

— 1989: *First language acquisition: method, description, and explanation*. Cambridge: Cambridge University Press.

INGRAM, D., CHRISTENSEN, L., VEACH, S. and WEBSTER, B. 1975: The acquisition of word initial fricatives and affricates in English by children between two and six. Research

Report, Child Language Project, Stanford University.

INGRAM, D. and TERSELIC, B. 1983: A case of deviant phonology. *Topics in Language Disorders* **3**, 45–50.

INTERNATIONAL PHONETIC ASSOCIATION 1949: *International Phonetic Alphabet*. London.

IRWIN, O. 1942: The developmental status of speech sounds of ten feeble-minded children. *Child Development* **13**, 29–39.

— 1947: Infant speech: consonantal sounds according to place of articulation. *JSHD* **12**, 397–401.

— 1951: Infant speech: consonantal position. *JSHD* **16**, 159–61.

JAKOBSON, R. 1968; *Child language, aphasia, and phonological universals*. The Hague: Mouton.

JAKOBSON, R. and HALLE, M. 1956: *Fundamentals of language*. The Hague: Mouton.

JESPERSEN, E. 1964: *Language: its nature, development, and origin*. New York: Norton.

JOHN, J.E. and HOWART, J.N. 1965: The effect of time distortions on the intelligibility of deaf children's speech. *Language and Speech* **8**, 127–34.

JOHNSON, C.E. and BUSH, C. 1971: A note on transcribing the speech of young children. *PRCLD* **3**, 95–100.

KAHN, L. 1986: *Basics of phonological analysis: a programmed learning text*. San Diego: College-Hill Press.

KARLIN, I.W. and STRAZZULA, M. 1952: Speech and language problems of mentally deficient children *JSHD* **17**, 286–94.

KORNFELD, J. 1971; Theoretical issues in child phonology. *PCLS*, Seventh Regional Meeting, 454–68.

LEONARD, L. 1985: Unusual and subtle phonological behavior in the speech of phonologically disordered children. *JSHD* **50**, 4–13.

LEONARD, L.B. 1973: The nature of deviant articulation. *JSHD* **38**, 156–61.

LEOPOLD, W. 1947: *Speech development of a bilingual child: a linguist's record* **2**. *Sound-learning in the first two years*. Evanston, Ill.: Northwestern University Press.

LEVITT, H. and SMITH, R. 1972: Errors of articulation in the speech of profoundly hearing-impaired children. *Journal of the Acoustical Society of America* **51**, 102–3.

LORENTZ, J. 1972: An analysis of some deviant phonological rules of English. Unpublished paper, University of California, Berkeley.

— 1974: A deviant phonological system of English. *PRCLD* **8**, 55–64.

LUKENS, H.T. 1894: Preliminary report on the learning of language. *Ped. Sem.* **3**, 424–60.

MACKEN, M.A. and FERGUSON, C.A. 1983: Cognitive aspects of phonological development: Model, evidence, and issues. In K.E. Nelson (ed.), *Children's language, Vol. 3*. Hillsdale, N.J.: Erlbaum, 256–82.

MARKIDES, A. 1970: The speech of deaf and partially-hearing children with special reference to factors affecting intelligibility. *British Journal of Disorders of Communication* **5**, 126–39.

MCCARTHY, D. 1930: *The language development of the preschool child*. Institute of Child Welfare, Monograph Series **4**. Minneapolis: University of Minnesota Press.

MCREYNOLDS, L. and BENNETT, S. 1972: Distinctive feature generalization in articulation training. *JSHD* **37**, 462–70.

MCREYNOLDS, L.V. and HUSTON, K. 1971: A distinctive feature analysis of children's misarticulations. *JSHD* **36**, 155–66.

MENN, L. 1971: Phonotactic rules in beginning speech. *Lingua* **26**, 225–51.

MENYUK, P. 1968: The role of distinctive features in children's acquisition of phonology. *JSHR* **11**, 138–46.

MENYUK, P. and LOONEY, P.L. 1972: Relationships among components of the grammar in language disorder. *JSHR* **15**, 395–406.

MILLER, J. and YODER, D. 1974: An ontogenetic language teaching strategy for retarded children. In Schiefelbusch and Lloyd, 505–28.

MILLER, P. 1972: Some context-free processes affecting vowels. In A. Zwicky (ed.), *Working Papers in Linguistics* **11**, 136–67, Ohio State University.

MOLL, K.L. 1968: Speech characteristics of individuals with cleft lip and palate. Chapter 3 in D. Spriesterbach and D. Sherman (eds.), *Cleft palate and communication*. New York: Academic Press.

MOORE, T. (ed.) 1973: *Cognitive development and the acquisition of language*. New York: Academic Press.

MOREHEAD, D. and INGRAM, D. 1973: The development of base syntax in normal and linguistically deviant children. *JSHR* **16**, 330–52.

MORLEY, M. 1957: *The development and disorders of speech in childhood*. London: Livingstone.

— 1966; *Cleft palate and speech*. Baltimore: Williams and Wilkins.

MORSE, P.A. 1974: Infant speech perception: a preliminary model and review of literature. In Schiefelbusch and Lloyd, 19–53.

MOSKOWITZ, A. 1970: The two-year-old stage in the acquisition of English phonology. *Language* **46**, 426–41.

— 1972; Review of Winitz: Articulatory Acquisition and Behavior. *Language* **48**, 487–98.

— 1973: On the status of vowel shift in English. In Moore (1973), 223–60.

NELSON, K. 1973: *Structure and strategy in learning to talk*. Monographs of the Society of Research in Child Development **38**, 1–2.

NEWMEYER, F. and EMONDS, J. 1971: The linguist in American society. *PCLS* Seventh Regional Meeting, 285–303.

NICE, M. 1925: Length of sentences as criterion of a child's progress in speech. *J. Educ. Psych* **16**, 370–9.

O'CONNOR, J.D. 1972: *Phonetics*. Harmondsworth, Middx: Penguin.

O'DONNELL, R.C., GRIFFIN, W.J. and NORRIS, R.C. 1967: *Syntax of kindergarten and elementary school children: a transformational analysis*. Champaign-Urbana, Ill.: National Council of Teachers of English.

OLLER, D.K. 1973: Regularities in abnorml child phonology. *JSHD* **38**, 36–47.

OLLER, D.K. *et al.* 1972; Five studies in abnormal phonology. Unpublished paper, University of Washington.

OLLER, D.K. and EILERS, R. 1975: Phonetic expectation and transcription validity. *Phonetica* (in press).

— (to be published): On phonology in hard-of-hearing children.

OLLER, D.K. and KELLY, C.A. 1974: Phonological processes of a hard-of-hearing child. *JSHD* **39**, 65–74.

OLLER, D.K., WEIMAN, L.A., DOYLE, W.J. and ROSS, C. 1974: Child speech, babbling, and phonological universals. *PRCLD* **8**, 33–41.

OLMSTED, D. 1971: *Out of the mouth of babes*. The Hague: Mouton.

— 1974; Review of N. Smith: The acquisition of phonology: a case study. *Journal of Child Language* **1**, 133–38.

PANAGOS, J. 1974: Persistence of the open syllable reinterpreted as a symptom of language disorder. *JSHD* **39**, 23–31.

PEIZER, D. and OLMSTED, D. 1969: Modules of grammar acquisition. *Language* **45**, 60–96.

PENDERGAST, R., DICKEY, S., SELMAR, J. and SODER, A. 1965: *Photo articulation test*. Chicago: King.

PHILIPS, B.J. and HARRISON, R.J. 1969: Articulation patterns of preschool cleft palate children. *The Cleft Palate Journal* **6**, 245–53.

PIAGET, J. 1955: *The language and thought of the child*. Cleveland: World Publishing Co.

— 1962: *Play, dreams, and imitation in childhood*. New York: Norton.

PIAGET, J. and INHELDER, B. 1969: *The psychology of the child*. New York: Basic Books.

POLLOCK, E. and REES, N. 1972; Disorders of articulation: some clinical applications of distinctive feature theory. *JSHD* **37**, 451–61.

POOLE, E. 1934: Genetic development of articulation of consonant sounds in speech. *Elementary English Review* **11**, 159–61.

PYE, C. and INGRAM, D. 1988: Automating the analysis of child phonology. *Clinical Linguistics and Phonetics* **2**, 115–37.

PYE, C., INGRAM, D. and LIST, H. 1987: A comparison of initial consonant acquisition in English and Quiché. In K.E. Nelson and A. Van Kleeck (eds.), *Children's language. Vol. 6.* Hillsdale, N.J.: Erlbaum, 175–90.

REES, N.S. 1973: Auditory processing factors in language disorders: the view from Procrustes' bed. *JSHD* **38**, 304–15.

RENFREW, C.E. 1966: Persistence of the open syllable in defective articulation. *JSHD* **31**, 370–73.

ROE, V. and MILISEN, R. 1942: The effect of maturation upon defective articulation in elementary grades. *JSHD* **7**, 37–50.

ROSS, A.S.C. 1937: An example of vowel-harmony in a young child. *Mod. Lang. Notes* **52**, 508–9.

SALUS, P.H. and SALUS, M.W. 1974: Developmental neurophysiology and phonological acquisition order. *Language* **50**, 151–60.

SANDER, E.K. 1961: When are speech sounds learned? *JSHD* **37**, 55–63.

SAX, M. 1972: A longitudinal study of articulation change. *J. Lang. Speech Hearing Serv. Schls.* **3**, 41–8.

SCHANE, S. 1973; *Generative phonology.* Englewood Cliffs, N.J.: Prentice-Hall.

SCHIEFELBUSCH, R. and LLOYD, L. (eds.) 1974: *Language perspectives—Acquisition, retardation, and intervention.* Baltimore: University Park Press.

SCHLANGER, B. 1953a; Speech measurements of institutionalized mentally handicapped children. *Amer. J. of Mental Deficiency* **58**, 114–22.

— 1953b: Speech examination of a group of institutionalized mentally handicapped children. *JSHD* **18**, 339–49.

SCHWARTZ, R. and LEONARD, L. 1982: Do children pick and choose? An examination of phonological selection and avoidance in early acquisition. *Journal of Child Language* **9**, 319–36.

SHRIBERG, L. and KWIATKOWSKI, J. 1980: *Natural process analysis (NPA).* New York: John Wiley.

SHRINER, T.H., HALLOWAY, M.S. and DANILOFF, R.G. 1969: The relationship between articulatory deficits and syntax in speech defective children. *JSHR* **12**, 319–25.

SHRINER, T., PRUTTING, C. and DANILOFF, R. 1970: Synergistic aspects of language performance. Unpublished paper, University of Illinois.

SHVACHKIN, N.K. 1973: The development of phonemic speech perception in early childhood. In C. Ferguson and D. Slobin (eds.), *Studies of child language development,* 91–127. New York: Holt, Rinehart, and Winston.

SMITH, M.W. and AINSWORTH, S. 1967: The effects of three types of stimulation on articulatory responses of speech defective children. *JSHR* **10**, 348–53.

SMITH, N. 1973: *The acquisition of phonology: a case study.* Cambridge: Cambridge University Press.

SNOW, K. and MILISEN, R. 1954: The influence of oral versus pictorial presentation upon articulation testing results. *JSHD,* Monograph Supplement, **4**, 29–36.

SPRIESTERBACH, D.C., DARLEY, F. and ROUSE, V. 1956: Articulation of a group of children with cleft lips and palates. *JSHD* **21**, 436–45.

STAMPE, D. 1969: The acquisition of phonetic representation. *PCLS,* 5th Regional Meeting, 443–54.

— 1972; A dissertation on natural phonology. Unpublished PhD dissertation, University of Chicago.

STOEL-GAMMON, C. and DUNN, C. 1985: *Normal and disordered phonology in children.* Baltimore, Md.: University Park Press.

STRAZULLA, M. 1953: Speech problems of the Mongoloid child. *Quarterly Review of Pediatrics* **8**, 268–73.

TEMPLIN, M. 1947: Spontaneous versus imitated verbalization in testing articulation in preschool children. *JSHD* **12**, 293–300.

— 1957: *Certain language skills in children: their development and interrelationships.* Institute of Child Welfare Monograph **26**. Minneapolis: The University of Minnesota Press.

TEMPLIN, M.C. and DARLEY, F.L. 1960: *The Templin–Darley tests of articulation.* Iowa City, Iowa: Bureau of Educational Research and Service, Extension Division, State University of Iowa.

TRACY, F. 1893: *The psychology of childhood.* Boston: Heath.

TYACK, D. and GOTTSLEBEN, R. 1974; *Language sampling, analysis and training.* Palo Alto, Cal.: Consulting Psychologists Press.

VELTEN, H. 1943: The growth of phonemic and lexical patterns in infant language. *Language* **19**, 281–92.

WATERSON, N. 1971: Child phonology: a prosodic view. *Journal of Linguistics* **7**, 170–221.

WEBER, J. 1970: Patterning of deviant articulation behavior. *JSHD* **35**, 135–41.

WEINER, F. 1979: *Phonological process analysis.* University Park Press: Baltimore, Md.

— 1981: Systematic sound preference as a characteristic of phonological disability. *JSHD* **46**, 281–6.

WELLMAN, B.L., CASE, I.M., MENGERT, I.G. and BRADBURY, D.E. 1931: Speech sounds of young children. *University of Iowa Studies in Child Welfare* **5**.

WEST, J.J. and WEBER, J.L. 1973: A phonological analysis of the spontaneous language of a four-year-old, hard-of-hearing child. *JSHD* **38**, 25–35.

WHITACRE, J.D., LUPER, H.L. and POLLIO, H.R. 1970: General language deficits in children with articulation problems. *Language and Speech* **13**, 231–9.

WINITZ, H. 1969: *Articulatory acquisition and behavior.* New York: Appleton-Century-Crofts.

Index

Cole & Whurr Journals of related interest

THE BRITISH JOURNAL OF DISORDERS OF COMMUNICATION

The British Journal of Disorders of Communication is an academically rigorous and intellectually challenging journal which presents the latest clinical and theoretical research and is a principal forum for the discussion of the entire range of communication disorders. The journal contains a representative and balanced selection of articles, with contributions from North America, Australasia and Continental Europe, as well as the UK. Among the leading articles published in recent issues are:
August 1987: Duncan & Gibbs - Acquisition of Syntax in Panjabi and English
December 1987: Gibbon and Hardcastle - Articulatory Description and Treatment of 'lateral /S/' using Electropalatography: A Case Study
April 1988: Perry - Surgical Voice Restoration following Laryngectomy: The Tracheo-oesophageal fistula technique (Singer-Blom)
August 1988: Bryan - Assessment of Language Disorders after Right Hemisphere Damage; Lebrun - Language and Epilepsy: A Review

The journal is owned by the College of Speech Therapists, and the Editor is Elspeth McCartney of Glasgow University and Jordanhill College. Issues are published three times a year and annual volumes are of up to 500 pages.

ISSN: 0007 098X

THE BRITISH JOURNAL OF EXPERIMENTAL AND CLINICAL HYPNOSIS

This is the Journal of the British Society of Experimental and Clinical Hypnosis, a learned society which brings together appropriately qualified medical professionals who have a legitimate reason for using hypnosis in their work and who share a scientific interest in the research and practical application of hypnosis. The journal provides a forum for the critical discussion of ideas, theories, findings, procedures and social policies associated with the topic of hypnosis. It also disseminates information on all aspects of theory, research and practice. A book review section is included.

ISSN:0265 1033

Please send for the Cole & Whurr catalogue.

Cole & Whurr Ltd
19b Compton Terrace, London N1 2UN
01-359 5979

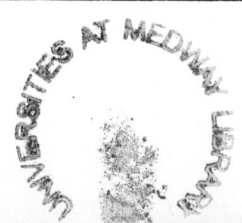